OLD–TIME

REMEDIES

For

Modern Ailments

OLD–TIME REMEDIES

For
Modern Ailments

by

Rev. Hanna Kroeger

About the Author

Hanna Kroeger, daughter of a German missionary, was born and raised in Turkey where she studied natural healing methods under the Oriental and European schools. After coming to the United States, she took advantage of the education offered by the American systems, ranging from Amerindian herbology to massage. She is an ordained minister in the Universal Church of the Masters, a church well known for its work in contact and spiritual healing. She is a nurse from Germany and has received her Doctorate of Metaphysics (MsD) from the State of Delaware. Besides teaching and lecturing, Mrs. Kroeger owns a health food store in Colorado and has for years owned and operated a health resort, the Peaceful Meadow Retreat, where she has seen her knowledge of nutrition used with exciting results.

This book is dedicated
to the wonderful people
of Boulder, Colorado.
God bless each one of you.

Rev. Hanna Kroeger

Contents

1. Fatigue and Lecithin.   1

2. About Fasting   7
   A. Rice Diet for Water-Logged Condition 12
   B. Fasting for Spiritual Reasons 13
   C. Three Days for Nerves 14
   D. Fasting for Kidney Ailments. 15
   E. Super Diet 16
   F. Cleansing Diet for the Liver, Pancreas and
      Upper Intestinal Tract. 19
   G. Reducing Diets. 21
   H. Fasting to Achieve Harmonization of the
      Digestive Tract. 22
   I. Fasting Replaces Sleep. 25
   J. Revitalizing Diet 26
   K. Clean Your Lymphatic System 28

3. Are Heavy Metals a Health Hazard?. 29
    A. Lead, Arsenic, Copper and Other Metal Poisoning . . 31
    B. Nickel 36
    C. Heavy Metal Reference 39

4. Magnetism. 41

5. Our Precious Youth 51

6. Metabolic Diseases and Enzymes. 57
    A. Enzymes: The Miracle Workers 59
    B. Ten-Day Regimen to Re-Establish
        Proper Enzyme Functioning 62

7. The Kidneys. 63

8. The Stomach 67

9. The Liver 75
    A. Apple Juice Diet. 77
    B. Liver Rejuvenating Recipes 79

10. The Lungs 81
    A. Lung Exercises. 86

11. Simian Virus 40 91

12. Old-Time Remedies 95
    A. Your Friends, the Friendly Bacteria 103

Introduction

Since the writing of this book in 1971, ever increasing numbers of men and women are becoming involved with natural foods and herbs. The movement is growing rapidly and making more important discoveries. Chemical and electromagnetic findings are of utmost interest for all of us.

In many hospitals, resorts and sanatoriums in Europe, both herbs and foods, as well as medicine, are used in perfect harmony and to the good of suffering mankind.

Remember, in no way will good, natural, nonchemical or unadulterated food and a cup of good herbal tea interfere with your physician's work. Your physician will be happy that you are more balanced—that you have more strength and endurance to weather long-time illnesses will delight him no doubt.

Fatigue and Lecithin

There is physically nothing wrong with you. Your heart beats its steady pace, your lungs are able to inhale deeply. Your blood is in good order. Kidneys are functioning and, yet, you push yourself with every step. Every task becomes a nightmare and just plain thinking is an effort, which you would rather put off until tomorrow. Fatigued, exhausted, depressed and so bitter and helpless against the nightmare of this experience. We have all had it at one time or another—after giving birth to a baby, after an operation or after a long, long sorrow. It comes with a hopeless-appearing situation. It is like a shadow monster which comes over you. You want to escape by sleeping but you wake up tired. You want to lick it by eating, however, after every meal you feel worse. You go to a movie, a dance, but you have to return early for want of rest. Pep pills make the situation worse in the long run and sleeping pills you don't need. You become a burden to your surroundings and friends and, in their eyes, you can see what they think. "Gosh, she is just pretending, there is nothing wrong with her."

We find the descriptions of fatigue in many old-time doctor books. I own one which was published in 1806 and in it it tells

1

the same story but they called it nerve fever, remarking that no fever is present. Strange name isn't it? We are more simplified and call it fatigue or exhaustion. The astounding part of this fatigue business is that even very young folks seem to suffer from fatigue. The effort to study or work seems too hard for them and their brain-fogged condition is due to fatigue.

Let's put some light on this problem. We are out of energy when our adrenal glands decide to provide us with less cortisone or when we have maltreated this perfectly good organ with too many no-no foods. Now there are very simple ways to give more specific food to this organ so that enough cortisone can be manufactured. The lowly alfalfa seed was used for centuries to battle fatigue. Soak three tablespoons alfalfa seed in one quart water overnight. Next morning bring to a boil and simmer for ten minutes. Drink as a breakfast drink with a little salt. Drink the rest without salt during the day. Blend two tablespoons sunflower seed and ten dates in one cup water. This restores energy beautifully. Lovely Mrs. Adelle Davis tells us that pantothenic acid and vitamin C are foods for the adrenal glands. Damiana leaves are a great help to restore nerve energies but one of the most important factors is lecithin.

What is lecithin? As far back as 1846, a chemist, M. Gabley, isolated a fat soluble substance from egg yolk which he called lecithin. Forty years later, Y. L. Thudichum found a similar substance in brain tissue which he called cephalin. Fifty years later, these findings were re-evaluated by two chemists, Schneider and Faleh. These chemists brought lecithin to the attention of the world. Lecithin is a compound of over seventy components. It belongs to the group of phosphatides because of its glycerin bound phosphorus.

Lecithin is found in plant life, as in seeds and yeast, and is particularly abundant in soybeans. It is found in animals. Blood cells, spinal cord and brain tissue are especially rich in lecithin. Organically raised eggs also have an abundance of lecithin. The human brain contains 28% lecithin and the spinal cord has not less than 25%. Every nerve is surrounded by a sheath which also contains 25% lecithin. Lecithin is abundant in heart tissue and the liver cannot function without it. Every cell wall has lecithin and

2

a network of lecithin is inside every cell wall. Here it is found in connection with protein, therefore, lecithin in this coalition is called lipoprotein.

Lecithin influences the structure of the protoplasm. It regulates the permeability of the cell walls. It is needed in carbohydrate, fat and protein digestion and is a balancing factor in the acid-alkalinity measure of the body. Lecithin, as mentioned, is needed for the metabolism of the nerve. That means no nerve vitality without lecithin. No wonder we are fatigued. Our body is not equipped to handle as much extra strain as our present mode of life prescribes. Unless we supply our chemistry with extra lecithin, extra choline and extra unsaturated fats, we cannot have the extra nerve pep we need.

The healthy body is able to make the different components for lecithin in the digestive tract and the liver. However, to bind, to tie these components together to form lecithin, we have to induce linoleic acid and choline. These two are the synergists, the spark that ties everything together to the compound called lecithin. That means that we have to have cold pressed oils and extra choline in our diets.

When should extra lecithin be taken and in what form? There is a crude oil on the market, cheap and terrible tasting and full of lecithin and linoleic acid. However, this lecithin is fat bound and not desirable for the emulsifying process of cholesterol. It is already fat bound and will not do you the favor of loosening its liaison to combine with the highly fat saturated cholesterol. The linoleic acid, however, will (if your intake of choline is sufficient) help you to form your own lecithin. Therefore, it is a preventive measure and should be evaluated only as such.

Lecithin in dry form was found accidentally during World War II when every ounce of fat had to be extracted for human consumption. This residue, as they thought it was, took on new dimensions in the industry. First, the chocolate industry got hold of it and found that this substance took care of the fat problem in their product without altering the taste. It emulsified the fats, so you were not aware that there was fat in chocolate, and made the product easier to digest. The candy industry was next and so the demand grew and grew. Now lecithin is one of the weapons

3

against high cholesterol, acting by emulsifying the fat in the body, veins and arteries, by supplying an easily digestible, easily absorbent choline. By introducing cephalin to the heart muscle, it helps against heart fatigue. The brain tissue is especially grateful for more cephalin in the diet. It also increases the peristaltic action of the intestines.

In 1952, Dr. Stefan found that injuries to the brain are greatly helped by lecithin. Patients with concussions and traumatic brain weaknesses improved in weeks instead of months when lecithin was given. It was given in a dry form.

We should assume that lecithin as it is, either in oil or granules, would be readily absorbed and utilized by the nervous system. It is so obvious when nerve exhaustion needs lecithin that lecithin should be given. However, both lecithin in crude oil form and lecithin in dry form have to undergo the enzymatic action of the digestive tract and cannot reach the crying nerves in these forms. Here you are. You know you need lecithin, your nerves are on edge, you are exhausted, fatigued, beaten down and your nerves cannot be reached in the simple way of eating lecithin granules or swallowing oil.

The enlightening work of Antom and Swanson brought light on this problem and gave us help and aid through their fabulous discoveries. They found that lecithin can be absorbed directly into the bloodstream if a lecithin molecule is smaller than a micron. They found a manufacturer who reduced the lecithin to a micro-differential, dispersible form and, guess what! The exhaustion problem was licked. The nerve food was found. Lecithin in this form does not have to undergo digestive enzymatic action but is carried right to the bloodstream and, from there, to the sheaths surrounding the nerves, the brain and the spinal cord.

We do not need case histories on this subject. All of us are exhausted at times without reason. Sleep does not restore our vitality, the cup of coffee seems to be the only pickup, just to let you sink deeper afterwards. Why not try the new exciting lecithin therapy? Our grandmother gave us egg yolks with honey but she watched that the yolks were dark orange. The light colored egg yolks were not used. I remember her buying calf brain for one of the members of the family and it was lightly steamed and served with orange colored raw egg yolks. I guess her common sense told her to feed lecithin for exhaustion and she had results. However, our mode of living has increased the need for lecithin tremendously and the orange colored egg yolks are not available any longer. So, thanks to the tremendous discoveries and the manufacturers, we get our lecithin nerve food on the market that will steady our nervous system, carry us over times of exhaustion and make every day of our lives worth experiencing.

Lecithin in oil—prevention.

Lecithin in granules—fat emulsifying.

Lecithin in microdifferential form—the new exciting nerve food.

Available as leciflow (lecithin with whey) or powdered lecithin.

About Fasting

About 2,500 years ago, Hippocrates, called the Father of Medicine, lived in Greece. His wisdom, his knowledge, his experiences were so outstanding that medicine of today still honors him. Hippocrates founded the humoral medicine and therapy which teaches that, whatever illness is expressed in a body, "look for difficulties in the fluids of the body." Study the "humors," the fluid. If you wish to improve the health of the body, everything should be done to improve the health of the humors.

Much later, in 1821-1902, came Virchow with his cellular medicine. The greatness and newness of his discovery shadowed the wisdom of Hippocrates. However, Hippocrates' followers were always active even when they were laughed at and persecuted. The theory and experience that sickness and illness cannot manifest in a healthy body and in a healthy blood and lymph stream has brought great scientists and great physicians to use their heads and work out plans for us laymen so that we may be able to prevent illness. Just as Hippocrates suggested, a healthy mind in a healthy body is now the goal of our new generation in America and all over the world. Prevention is the goal and preventive medicine was originated by Hippocrates.

The human body consists of more than nine-tenths fluid. Some of the fluid is bound in the cells and is a substance of the cell. Some of the fluid, as lymph fluid, blood fluid and juices of the hormone cycle, are outside of the cells and bathe the cells, so to speak, from the outside. According to the different tasks of the humors (which means fluids), they have different appearances and different colors: light red, dark red, transparent, milky, etc. Because of the fluidic and moving state of these different "humors," it stands to reason that they interchange and exchange with each other and that they also permeate every cell and every organ of the living body.

There is no doubt that different organs finally break down when a continuous stream of unhealthy, undernourished and impoverished fluids surrounds and penetrates them. "Nutrients being preserved with chemicals will stay preserved to a large percentage in the body," Professor Brauchle warned.

Nutrition overloaded with sweets will weaken the humoral fluid greatly. Nutrients lacking in minerals will not restore nor prevent anything. The loss of minerals in some fluids, as urine, saliva and perspiration, has to be made up daily.

We have four to five quarts of blood and about two quarts of lymph fluid. We produce in twenty-four hours one and one half quarts saliva, two and one half quarts stomach juices, one quart gall and three quarts intestinal juices. All of these fluids end up in the intestinal tract. From here they are reabsorbed and purified and return to be reused. Only about two to three quarts leave the body daily and this has to be replaced daily. If we continually replace these missing fluids with soda water, Coca-Cola, sugar syrups and other nonnutritional hoaxes, we soon will reap what we have been sowing.

What is fasting? Fasting is a willful abstinence from solid foods, and sometimes also liquids, which is done for a specific purpose. Fasting has been done since mankind existed. Many passages in the Bible show us that, in Biblical times, people used fasts. These people used it mainly for spiritual reasons. They prepared themselves to walk with the Lord by conquering the carnal man and practiced it in periodic fasting.

Many religions have maintained strict rules over the centuries about food intake and occasional fasting. For example, there is the Islam whose followers never touch pork, maybe because of the danger of possible trichinosis. They are also forbidden to drink alcoholic beverages. The Catholic church still keeps the Lent season and their followers abstain from meat and sweets for several weeks. As time marched on, people found out that fasting is not only meant for religious reasons but, by willfully staying away from solid foods, their will power increased. Many powerful leaders of nations, religions and societies make a point in abstaining from food for several days at a time, just to clarify their thinking, to increase their will power and to become better men.

Fasting is not starvation. Starvation is a slow process of painful dying while the body consumes itself. "With starvation you become a meat eater by eating, digesting, consuming your own body," Dr. Carlton Federicks stated.

I had the privilege and the great fortune to have known Professor Brauchle, a man of great foresight and love, who directed a 1,200 bed hospital in Dresden, now East Germany. Most of the patients were treated with natural methods: baths, fasting, diets, therapeutic massage, herbs and vitamins alone. Some of them were treated, in addition to natural methods, with allopathic procedures. The most happy combinations, however, were when Professor Brauchle started to employ men and women who sat down with the patient to discuss their inner problems. These workers strengthened the will power of the patient, helped them to overcome doubts and difficulties, hate and destructive thoughts and reestablished hope and peace.

In his interesting and famous lectures, Professor Brauchle taught us that fasting is equal to a surgeon's knife. It does away with accumulated toxins of all kinds. In his lectures he told of case history after case history where, under scientific, supervised fasting, people returned to perfect health. He continued to say that raw food diet is the weapon of a physician for internal medicine and that a mixed diet is for the working man.

9

Now, if fasting is a physician's knife, we have to ask ourselves what is wrong with us that we want to have corrected. A surgeon does not perform an appendectomy when he wants to take out tonsils. He uses different methods for different purposes. A fast, therefore, must be directed to the purpose in a correct manner. Just to say "I am staying away from food" is neither purposeful nor scientific. Therefore, when you want to undergo a fast, ask yourself, "What do I want to achieve? Do I want to get rid of a certain affliction? Do I want to walk closer with God? Do I want to lose weight? What do I want?"

Mankind has invented many fasts. The Turks fast on delicious watermelons once a year; the Bulgarians on yogurt. The Romans drank the mineral spring water. These old-time fasts are not scientific and are undertaken more or less because of tradition, just as grandmother gave sulfur and molasses every spring to every member of the family. If needed or not, everyone got his spoonful of molasses twice a day for a week or more. We have to become scientific and specific when it comes to fasting. It must be purposeful and meaningful. It must help your body and not destroy your body. It must support the effort your physician puts out for you. It should be done only for a short period and in full acceptance with your inner self.

I am giving you several time proven, purposeful, scientific fasts which are mainly used in Europe and administered in the clinics of famous physicians.

A fast on water alone, as it was done and advocated thirty years ago, was safe and effective. Not so today. In our fatty tissue all of us have accumulated DDT and other matter. A water fast loosens these foreign accumulations but, instead of throwing them through the liver into the intestine, they are driven into the bone marrow. This is the last place you want poisons to accumulate.

Dr. Buchinger, a man who fasted thousands of people with great success, uses the following method: fresh pressed juices. This means freshly pressed fruits or vegetables. The juice must be diluted with water, half and half, or you may drink one glass juice and one glass water at the same time. This is greatly used in:

infectious diseases
hypertension
leg ulcers
kidney disorders
skin diseases
rheumatic diseases

When you do it yourself, never do it longer than four days at a time and only once or twice a month if needed. Never use fruit and vegetable juices at the same time. You may alternate them. Always take one or two enemas a day if undertaking a juice fast.

One requisite is to take it easy during a fast. If you can afford it, stay only half days on your job or take the first part of your vacation for this purpose. Secondly, don't feel sorry for yourself. Your food will taste better afterwards and you will feel so good just because you conquered the carnal man in you. Before you start a fast, consign your mind to it. Don't you make up your mind before you undergo an operation? Surely you do and you know some parts of it are not so pleasant. Just feel yourself being wheeled into the operating room, the very thought of it gives everyone the chills. Some parts of fasting are not so pleasant either, particularly the first three days when the poisons loosen from the subcutaneous tissue. But again, the first three days after an operation are not so pleasant either. In any case, make up your mind and no uncle, aunt, neighbor or anyone else should change your opinion. The best is not to tell anyone, just do it!

A. Rice Diet for Water-Logged Condition

Take one cup brown rice (short grain is to be preferred because it has more minerals). Wash it and put it in two cups boiling water without salt. Boil for thirty-five minutes on low heat. This kind of rice is to be eaten whenever one is hungry. At noon and night some applesauce or stewed pears without sugar might be added. Or you may boil some wheat germ and middlings in water and use as you would the above recipe. For best results, do it five to seven days.

How and why does this diet work? When the sodium, which is in the fluid surrounding the cell, comes in disharmony with the potassium, which is supposed to be in the cell, fluid builds up. The fluid is kept in proper proportion and harmony through the positive and negative electricity of the two opponents and components, sodium and potassium. When the sodium decides to pay a visit to the potassium in the cell, the potassium will leave. The sodium, which has no business in the cell, cannot handle the incoming fluid and you start to be water-logged.

B. Fasting for Spiritual Reasons

Fasting for spiritual reasons is practiced widely by our precious youth. It is a fad, unfortunately, an ego trip for many to fast senselessly for prolonged periods of time. They go on water, the worst they can do, and overdraw their capacity of fasting to the point of delayed return or even no return. Please, young people, listen. Do not go on water fasts. The short cut to fasting for spiritual reasons is the following approved method. It is very, very effective.

Take one pound manukka raisins and soak them in four quarts water, distilled preferred, for twenty-four hours. Stir frequently and drink one to one and one-half quarts of the water in small sips in the morning from 7 a.m. to 11 a.m. or 8 a.m. to noon. For one hour take neither food nor drink and have lunch consisting of vegetable and salad with fish, eggs or cheese. The supper is your choice of food but should not be taken later than 6 p.m. Do this for two to four weeks, or as you feel it is necessary. Meditate short periods, five to ten minutes, several times a day. It is not the length, it is the depth that counts for us Westerners.

You may also use thirty-six ounces of grape juice in the above described manner, however, you have to add six ounces of water to the thirty-six ounces of grape juice in order for it to work. Why? I don't know. It must be a secret of the electromagnetic field which we do not know too much about.

C. Three Days for Nerves

It takes will power and authority to stay on a diet, especially when your nerves give out.

Following routine only three days in a row will make a better "boss," a stronger personality out of you. After that, one day a week or one day every two weeks will keep your nerves sweet.

In one pint of cottage cheese mix three tablespoons almond oil or safflower oil and two egg yolks. Mix well and either make it sweet with honey or spicy with onions, salt and herbs. Also boil four tablespoons of barley in two quarts water for thirty-five minutes. Strain and add honey and lime or lemon juice to the barley water so it tastes good.

Before breakfast: one cup of warm barley water
Breakfast: prepared cottage cheese; carrots, raw or cooked
Mid-morning: barley water
Noon: steamed zucchini; cooked green beans; cottage cheese, spicy
Mid-afternoon: barley water
Evening: cottage cheese; zucchini, stewed or baked in the oven; dish of barley; carrot salad; barley water
Bedtime: barley water; calcium tablets

D. Fasting for Kidney Ailments

Boil crushed watermelon seeds, one cup to three quarts water, for three minutes. Strain and store two quarts in refrigerator while leaving the rest on the table. Every hour take one-third cup of this lukewarm tea. For breakfast take watermelon. For lunch take acidophilus milk and/or yogurt, vegetable and raw food, some fish or egg and rye bread. Supper is stewed pears or applesauce with yogurt or soy milk, as much as you like. Do this diet for three days but continue watermelon seed tea and watermelon breakfasts for fourteen days.

This recipe comes from Turkey. It was given to my mother by a prominent religious authority. I have given away this recipe many times. Every time the result was immediate and astounding. It balances the fluids in the system by releasing electrical currents and re-establishing the yin-yang function of the kidney.

E. Super Diet

Clay for healing has been used since mankind existed. Even the Bible tells us how Jesus took clay for healing the sick and as a medium of his divine power.

The mud baths used in European health spas are famous. These special clays or muds are full of natural hormones and vitamins E, A and B-complex. There are thankful women who, after taking a series of baths, return to health and youth singing praises to mud treatments.

In Europe, Luvas Healing Earth "Heilerde" is sold in drugstores. Every household has it in its medicine cabinet. For upset stomachs these people take one-half teaspoon in one glass of water. For diarrhea they take one teaspoon in one-half glass of water. For food poisoning they take it every half hour. For sore feet they put it in the foot bath water. For skin eruptions they make a thin paste and apply that. In our hospital (Dresden) we use it on old sores. We just powdered them with clay dust.

Volcanic ash is a cheap and versatile home remedy. It was first used on a great scale by the British army. During the Balkan War, mortality from cholera was terrific. Sixty percent of all soldiers who contracted this disease died. When solutions of volcanic ash were introduced, the mortality rate went down to three percent. Since that, the British army uses clay for the treatment of acute food poisoning.

How does volcanic ash work? According to leading experts on geology, volcanic ash has one of the world's smallest molecules. These molecules are shaped like calling cards. The two broad surfaces have a negative electrical attraction while the edges are positive. Therefore, volcanic ash can pick up many times its own weight of positive charged ions. Certain toxins and bacteria found at times in the body, and in the alimentary tract in particular, are of positive charge. Volcanic ash absorbs or neutralizes such intruders and, in this way, volcanic ash aids in the detoxification of the alimentary canal. It took an ingenious American man to realize these facts and to have the foresight to bring a product on the market which everyone can use in confidence and to full benefit. Mr. Irons took volcanic ash and emulsified it in a truly ingenious way. His product stays in suspension and does not settle to the bottom of the bottle.

Experiments of Dr. Howard E. Lind, on the subject of hydrated water suspended bentonite (volcanic ash), are extremely fascinating. They bring into scientific terms what our forefathers knew by experience. In his laboratory Dr. Lind experimented with volcanic ash. He placed 4,095,000 bacteria count in a medium and covered it with hydrated bentonite. After sixty minutes the count was reduced to 2,495,000. After ninety minutes there were only 620,000 left. He made many other experiments with equal success and found that volcanic ash even neutralizes the dreaded staph bacillus.

Whenever the problem of health is partially or totally due to a toxic, overloaded alimentary tract, this scientific and, therefore, very effective fast on volcanic ash should be considered. Here it is:

> take two to three tablespoons of liquid bentonite in one glass water
> take one heaping teaspoon of detox or psyllium seed or intestinal cleanser (a bulk making item) in one glass unsweetened juice
> drink more fluids, like herb tea or water, after so that you have a total fluid intake of sixteen ounces

Do this five times a day: at 7 a.m., 10 a.m., 1 p.m., 4 p.m. and 7 p.m. At 9 p.m. take an enema to eliminate all the waste from your colon so you may sleep soundly. On the fourth or fifth day you will lose, besides long ropes of waste, black matter which is the sign that you may start adding food to your diet like some raw and steamed vegetables and raw and steamed fruit. Discontinue clay after the seventh day, re-establish friendly bacteria with acidophilus or yogurt and go on a good, natural diet.

This fast is modern. It is without hunger pangs. It is effective and helpful and cooperates beautifully with your physician's suggestions. In case you need an operation, it is much easier for a surgeon to work when the alimentary tract is free of old waste. I know by experience as a nurse on the instrument tables how unhappy surgeons are when an overloaded "wastebasket" alimentary tract hinders and holds up proper surgical procedures.

Some time ago, I talked to an undertaker to find out what his side of the big tragedy was and what he had to contribute to help mankind. His biggest concern was the putrefaction of the alimentary canal. He said there are people with sixty pounds of waste in their intestine. They choked to death, he said.

That did it. The next morning I went on the clay diet. I was not hungry at all and worked all day long feeling happier and happier. On the third day the stool looked like long ropes of old waste, rubber like and terrible. The old pockets had been emptying. Stuff sitting there for years and glued to the intestinal walls loosened out. Most probably the white gluten bread I used for two years had baked to the intestinal walls. Since that, twice a year I go on a three-day clay diet just to have my intestinal tract in the best shape possible.

Mrs. R. told me her story and experience on this matter. She was fifty-four years old when it started. She complained of pain in her legs. Since she was somewhat on the heavy side, all tests were made for diabetes and similar ailments. She stopped smoking, lived on diet products for losing weight and got worse and worse. A year later the right leg was blue and discolored and both legs were swollen and painful—no circulation. After six more months of intense suffering, amputation of the right leg was suggested. Someone had told her about the healing clay and Mrs. R. started the very same day. For seven days the old waste, accumulated from years of constipation, poured out. With every day she felt stronger. On her seventh day the pain in her legs was gone. There was still some swelling and discoloration, she said, but she could walk. So she walked to the dress shop and shoe store to buy herself a new outfit for a new lease on life.

F. Cleansing Diet for the Liver, Pancreas and Upper Intestinal Tract

First on arising: one-half grapefruit (if hungry)
Breakfast: all the cooked or canned whole tomatoes you wish
Mid-morning: one whole grapefruit
Noon meal: same as breakfast
Mid-afternoon: one whole grapefruit
Dinner meal: same as noon meal
Bedtime: one-half grapefruit (if hungry)

Eat nothing but the above for four to seven days, depending on the conditions or poison. This is very good and should not disturb the patient. In some cases this diet will bring on a fever as the body starts to throw off the poison. This is also good and should not disturb the patient.

World famous Dr. Evers, whose diet reform brings many multiple sclerosis patients back to health and to walking, does this almost with diet alone. He teaches his patients how to sprout wheat and rye. His patients can eat these sprouts twice a day. He gives them hazelnuts, walnuts, sunflower seed, coconut, Brazil nuts, raw eggs and raw milk. For fresh fruits he gives them apples, pears, plums, cherries and all berries. For sweets the patients can have raisins, dates and figs. For vegetables Dr. Evers gives only those that grow under the ground, as carrots, radishes, red beets, etc. For starches he gives whole wheat, rye bread and raw rolled oats. With this diet, which is full of life enzyme, a drastic change in the sluggish metabolism is achieved and Dr. Evers has results. To begin:

For liver only:

First day, on arising, drink eight ounces of hot water with fresh lemons squeezed into it. From then on drink the juice for breakfast, lunch, dinner and whenever hungry. Also, stewed tomatoes and tomato juice may be taken, as it is also a cleanser. Drink hot water and lemon or tomato juice whenever you feel like it, the more the better. Do not worry about the following day because it is the same procedure.

It is amazing how hungry you become so, at bedtime of the second day, you will look forward to the following cocktail:

three ounces olive oil
two ounces castor oil
three ounces whip cream

Be ready for sleep and be relaxed. Drink before bed and you may chew a little piece of lemon afterwards, just for taste. It is a lot easier than it sounds! At 3 or 4 a.m., you will be having a nature's call and, in all your life, you have not experienced so much dark and ugly smelling waste. The next morning have a breakfast you desire and earned!

Stewed tomatoes: Take ripe tomatoes and cut out the place where the stem is because this part of the plant is not fit to eat and, in most cases, is poisonous. Tomatoes belong to the berry family and you can core out the stem from strawberries too. Cut tomatoes in little pieces, add a little water and simmer them slowly. You may add salt, onions or seasoning but no fat of any kind.

G. Reducing Diets

A severe overweight condition is a big problem. You have to have help from your physician. Here are some suggestions:

A) When you are too round around the middle, follow Dr. Ellis' diet: B_6 and magnesium gluconate, safflower oil and high protein.
B) If your thighs are too heavy, avoid all sweets for good. Have more gland food such as liver, sprouts, vitamins E, B_1 and B-complex.
C) If you are too heavy all around, try Gaylord Hauser's Fourteen Day Rejuvenation Diet. Count calories and drink a tea made of chickweed, burdock and nettle brewed for twenty minutes.
D) When water-logged, try wheat germ and middlings for one week. Also use vitamins E and C which act as diuretics and are treasured by many people for this property.

For people who are sensitive to their environment and the negative force fields of others, it is advisable to protect themselves from destruction by putting on some weight. It certainly helps a lot.

H. Fasting to Achieve Harmonization of the Digestive Tract

Dr. Mayr, Germany, invented a truly genuine procedure of fasting. His theory is that, in order to have health, your digestive tract has to be in good shape. He said that no food, no vitamin, no mineral can properly be utilized in the body unless the digestive tract is functioning well. The intestine has to work harmoniously.

Here is his fasting regimen, which should be carried on for about four to six weeks. One can do it during vacation or in a resort but many do it while working full-time. I must say it is astoundingly easy and unusually effective. Ask your baker to supply you with hard rolls. If you don't have a bakery, make your own. Let these rolls sit for one day or until they become ready to cut without crumbling. Again, the rolls should not be too dry, which would interfere with your program. For the success of this fasting, it is important to have the right consistency of the rolls. Not fresh and not too dry. You start your day with a light solution of Epsom salts water. Take one teaspoon Epsom salts in four ounces water and drink slowly. You cut your rolls in small pieces and chew each piece very thoroughly and long, until it is liquefied and becomes sweet. Now you spoon one teaspoon milk or buttermilk and swallow it down. Then take the next piece of roll and continue until you are really satisfied. It is amazing how long this meal stays with you. You are not hungry at all until noon, then you do the very same thing. In between meals drink herbal teas, such as chamomile, linden blossom, peppermint or any other tea with a little honey. At night you eat rolled oats blended through a sieve, or wheat prepared the same way, and eat your rolls with sips of milk. Never drink milk alone even when you have some left over in your cup. This would bloat you and disturb the bacteria you are trying to rebuild in your intestinal tract. Every day take the juice of one lemon or one orange to supply you with vitamin C and trace elements. After the stool begins to have a golden color and is odorless (about one to two weeks), you add one soft-boiled egg, some butter, cottage cheese and some creamed soup but let these be additions to the fundamental roll and milk diet.

Dr. Mayr knows that this regimen is lacking in protein and vitamins but do not be disturbed by this. A sick digestive tract cannot digest the best food you place in it. It only makes gas, putrefaction and deposits (because it is so weak). Everything settles in the pockets, curves and folds of the tract. So first re-establish the proper functioning of the colon and you will be satisfied with the end result.

Mrs. Clark, fifty years of age, appeared to be much older. Her abdomen was protruding heavily. Her skin looked grey and wrinkled. She had a double chin and her exhaustion was visible and expressed in every movement she made. All her life she was on laxatives, sometimes four to six a day, but very poor results were obtained. Mrs. Clark started Dr. Mayr's method in a German clinic and returned four weeks later to the USA a different woman. Gone was the double chin. Gone was the protruding abdomen. No more laxatives. She appeared ten years younger. She continued to improve and, by Christmas, her skin was almost wrinkle free.

Mr. X always had trouble with bloatedness after meals. His gallbladder had been removed some years ago but to no avail. The trouble with gas, irregularity and a sickish feeling remained and he was about to sell his business in order to retire at too early an age. When he heard about Dr. Mayr's diet, he at once submitted to it and the result was phenomenal. A cranky, sickly person was converted to a robust, healthy man in a matter of a few weeks.

Carol was a saleslady in a ready wear department. She was very good and efficient, however, she got fired because of her skin problem which no makeup could hide. Penicillin, Terramycin and streptomycin only brought temporary relief and, later, big pus filled blisters appeared all over her body. Carol was desperate and her decision was suicide. When she heard about Dr. Mayr's diet regimen, she just jumped at it because she had no money for food and this seemed practical and inexpensive. She got better and, after six weeks, took on a very well paid job as a department manager. Her skin became more beautiful with every day and continued looking nicer long after she discarded the monotonous diet. However, once a year she goes back on it for three to four weeks which is her skin and health secret.

How does Dr. Mayr's diet work?

a) It re-establishes friendly bacteria;
b) it lubricates every morsel put in the mouth;
c) it relaxes the nerves of the intestinal tract;
d) it takes out accumulated poisons; and
e) it harmonizes the intestinal tract.

Dr. Mayr stated that, in many people, parts of the intestinal tract work too fast. Others are spastic, other parts may be clogged with waste and still others work normally. The harmonization of the intestinal tract also will be expressed in the harmonization of the human individual. From a cranky, sickly, complaining man or woman rises a phoenix of beauty and harmony.

I. Fasting Replaces Sleep

Whenever you have to miss sleep, drink acidophilus culture. It comes in pint bottles. Take one-half cup several times a day with very, very little raw food, just to satisfy your stomach nerves and muscles. Increasingly you will feel better and better. Whenever you can sleep again, your sleep will be normal in length and you will wake up refreshed as always. Since this book is written in my spare time between two jobs, I can verify this method myself. Sometimes I get carried away and work through my sleeping hours. Acidophilus replaces my sleep and makes thinking clear.

J. Revitalizing Diet

After eating a lifetime of wrong food combinations poisoned by chemicals, additives and no energy, your body rebels. Nothing works any longer. The eyes give out. Everything hurts. The blood pressure plays escalator (up and down with every mood). The heart pounds and shortness of breath begins. In short, you are going to pieces! Now is the time to think of doing something fundamental, something that will change your life, something that turns the ship around!

Saturday morning make your decision for one week and two days and these will be the best nine days of your life.

7 a.m.	four ounces sauerkraut juice
	four ounces tomato juice
8 a.m.	six to seven ounces hot lemon juice
9 a.m.	six to seven ounces hot vegetable broth
10 a.m.	six to seven ounces cool grapefruit juice
11 a.m.	six to seven ounces hot vegetable broth
12 p.m.	large green salad with dressing of vinegar, sea salt, oil and spices; cucumber and tomato slices allowed
1 p.m.	six to seven ounces cool grapefruit juice
2 p.m.	six to seven ounces vegetable broth
3 p.m.	six to seven ounces cool lemonade
4 p.m.	six to seven ounces hot vegetable broth
5 p.m.	six to seven ounces cool grapefruit juice
6 p.m.	vegetable salad as at noon
7 p.m.	six to seven ounces hot vegetable broth
8 p.m.	yogurt or buttermilk or juice

If you need a laxative, then take it at bedtime. You should have good bowel action. Every third day make the following enema (exception: not when you are a diabetic):

One quart of water and three-quarters cup honey—mix well.

And in the morning, whenever you have time, cleanse your system with it.

This diet of hot and cold (please, no ice), of salty and sweet (grapefruit juice), stimulates the complete defense mechanism of your body. The tissue will let go with the accumulated waste material. The bowels will empty and the pancreas and liver will make house cleaning. The brain starts throwing out the cobwebs and lymph and blood will be rejuvenated.

I suggest you take a little cabin somewhere away from temptation and suggestions of your friends and enjoy the return of your health.

K. Clean Your Lymphatic System

    one pint white grapefruit juice
    one pint freshly squeezed orange juice
    one pint grape juice
    one pint water with the juice of three limes
    one pint water with the juice of two lemons
    one pint frozen pineapple juice, diluted
    one pint papaya juice, diluted
    twelve eggs (whole)
    six egg yolks
    frozen raspberries or strawberries add a delicious flavor
    beat eggs and mix into fruit juice mixture

This is one day's supply. If you are hungry add one kind of fresh fruit. For lunch, green salad and/or sprouts with raw almond dressing. For supper, green salad and/or sprouts with raw almond dressing and one steamed vegetable.

Are Heavy Metals a Health Hazard?

At the University of Erlangen, a team of scientists examined 158 steel workers and garbage collectors for lead residue in their systems. These people remain in the streets which are full of car exhaust for over eight hours a day and have to breathe the lead of the car exhaust more than any other citizens. It was found that the d-aminolavulin acid levels in the urine and blood of these 158 men were extremely high. Twenty-six of these men were, in medical respect and diagnosis, unable to work since the fallout of car exhaust had elevated the d-aminolavulin acid dangerously high, showing an acute lead poisoning. These twenty-six men all complained of exhaustion but showed no other physical signs. Apparently, the body had compensated somehow for the ever increasing lead residue in the system. The question here is how much lead does the average person have and how much longer will the system compensate until it breaks down with a bang?!

It is said that the fall of Rome was nothing more than the accumulated lead poisoning in their citizens. They used to carry their water in lead pipes and lead containers and the accumulated lead destroyed the nation. Our water pipes are safe but how about the air we breathe? Are the cities and crowded highways safe?

On windless days you see the car exhausts lingering over our highways. In a long stripe of grey-blue, it lies there like a monster. In fact, it is a monster which eats up our health. When lead is taken in through the lungs, it is more likely to be in suspension in the fluids of the body, like the lymphatic, blood and gland fluids. When eaten with food, as the Romans did, it is more likely to be deposited in the joints, liver, pancreas and heart.

The Biologisch-physicalische Research Institute in Obergensingen, West Germany, reports that the lead contamination of the atmosphere is increasingly alarming. Every fourth patient shows lead poisoning. Most probably the car exhaust is at fault in this misery. Every gallon of gasoline contains sixty milligrams of lead. Approximately 8,000 tons of this metal is puffed into the atmosphere every year. In the streets, children and small animals are particularly exposed to the dangers of poisons through heavy metal accumulations in the atmosphere, since these metals have a tendency to settle down.

The scientists of Obergensingen developed an instrument which enables them to test 1,000 blood samples a day. Desperately, they try to find the antidote to the accumulations of lead residue in humans and animals. Their findings are widely publicized to change the condition of air pollution, at least in their country.

A. Lead, Arsenic, Copper and Other Metal Poisoning

Lead is a protoplasmic poison which means that it interferes with the proper life-energy-enzyme exchange in the living body. It is amazing how beautifully our system is able to take this load of lead poisoning. Everyone has it. Only a few people in very isolated places in the mountains or prairies are free from lead intoxication.

There is to be considered: the amount of lead in our system; the tolerance factor of lead, arsenic, cadmium, mercury, copper and other heavy metals. This tolerance factor differs in everyone. Some people sponge in more arsenic than others, some sponge in more lead or aluminum or mercury. I found redheaded people are prone to take in more copper than others. And orientals take in more mercury. The fair people take in more lead and aluminum. The individual tolerance also differs widely. In every case of leukemia, the tolerance level of arsenic should be checked. In every case of exhaustion, the lead level should be checked. In every case of numbness, sore mouth and gums, the mercury level should be checked.

Here is a typical pattern of complaint: A young mother, happily married, complains of "tired blood," irritability, listlessness. She goes to the drugstore to get some iron tonic but it does not help. Three weeks later, she complains of exhaustion. She consults a physician and he helps her with pep pills but now sleeplessness and exhaustion set in. She now takes tranquilizers in the evening and the pep pills in the morning. The nervous system revolts and marriage problems set in. Crying spells or rage, depending on temperaments, become a daily scene. The psychiatrist suggests that she has housewife syndrome and should go find a part-time job. However, this does not work either and employers become unhappy with her. Finally, it is suggested that her marriage is a failure and the judge has to decide what to do next.

And all the complaints because of metal intoxication.

Here is another one: The little three-year-old becomes increasingly listless. She has no appetite, food is tasteless to her. She lays on the floor sucking her thumb, one of her little hands stroking a toy over and over again. Blood tests show nothing. When you touch her she cries as if in pain, particularly when you pull her up by grasping her hands or her shoulders. The nights are restless and she has nightmares. Her brother just entered school and mother is happy to have this loud, noisy kid out of her hair. Every toy of his is broken, he constantly picks on the little girl, he has no discipline. But after four weeks, a note from the teacher arrives that John has to be taken to the physician or a tranquilizer has to be given to him in school. A first start for a drug addiction later in life.

These are two stories you find over and over again and every schoolteacher has seen these two types. Both are metal intoxicated, both are sick, both are in need of help at once. The parents are the only ones who can help. The government cannot help, your physician cannot help. He does not cook the meals. He is not your nutritionist. You are the only one who can do something about it. Here are some recipes for you:

        one gallon cranberry juice
        three tablespoons whole cloves
        two teaspoons ground cinnamon
        one teaspoon cream of tartar

Boil the cloves in one quart cranberry juice for twenty minutes. Strain and add two teaspoons ground cinnamon. Stir and add it to the rest of the cranberry juice. Now add one teaspoon cream of tartar. Stir. Drink five ounces three times daily. For children, three ounces three times daily for twelve to fifteen days. Then do it once a week. In case lead or other heavy metals are lodged in the joints and it pains you, the following recipe will help. It comes from the Romans.

Take a soft piece of leather and spread a pulp of comfrey root on it. Apply this to the suffering joints every night.

A wonderful herbal formula for taking out lead residue is:

        six ounces basil
        one ounce rosemary
        one ounce hyssop
        one ounce boneset

Mix these, make a tea and drink one cup three times daily.

In Germany, they found that red cabbage counteracts lead poisoning when lead is in humoral suspension which means when lead is not lodged but suspended in the fluids of the body.

There is an old Roman manuscript found which received lots of attention in the 1930s. I heard of it when I was working as a public health nurse in Germany. Our physician in charge was great in natural remedies and discussed some of his findings and the manuscript in lectures with us. Here is what the Romans did. They dried okra and made a powder from it. They also ground pumpkin seeds and mixed both together. They added a little cayenne pepper and took some of this mixture in rhubarb sauce. I tried it and it is fabulous, as in the following proportions:

two tablespoons pumpkin seeds, ground
one tablespoon okra powder
one-half teaspoon cayenne pepper

When mixed, I take one teaspoon of this in some rhubarb sauce (one tablespoon) about three times a day for ten days.

One of the most universal remedies to remove lead, arsenic, platinum, gold and mercury from your body are sulfur baths. The sulfur baths in Europe are overcrowded. Many Americans find help there. Every summer a stream of Americans fly to European spas to take care of their problems with health. We have these wonderful healing waters right here in this country. They are undiscovered and unattended. The precious water runs away into the beautiful wilderness. A national campaign should be started to build beautiful spas around these precious sulfur waters of America. It should be made available to rich and poor alike.

Thanks to the advancement of industry, sulfur baths are available in dry form and the granules or tablets or powders can be added to the bath water. When we take it by mouth, sulfur is easily overdosed but, in bath, the body takes in only what it needs. Once a month, particularly for women after menstruation, a sulfur bath is good. At that time, the female needs a small amount of sulfur to form the proper amino acid combination to further carry on proper nutrition for the reproductive organs.

33

Dr. Hazel Parcells, thank God for her love to mankind, came up with a most unique and most modern way to counteract heavy metal deposits. She puts seven ounces Clorox in a good sized bathtub and tells people to stay in this warm bath for ten to fifteen minutes. What a relief to our nerves! What a blessing she puts into every home. Rinse your skin carefully afterwards. Warning: Not everyone can take Clorox baths. We find some super allergic people have a bad reaction. In order to find out who can take it and who cannot, make a weak, warm solution (one teaspoon Clorox to one gallon of warm water) and wash your feet in it. Children do well with foot baths as described.

Herbs that contain a lot of sulfur are watercress, eyebright, nettle, fennel, mullein and coltsfoot. These herbs, when eaten fresh, are more effective in supplying natural sulfur than when dried and brewed. Do they help to counteract lead poison? I do not know. I just give them so you may have something to think about.

Copper poisoned people have a burning sensation in throat and tonsils and some have it all through the system. The copper poisoned individual wants to open his hands all the time. I have seen people opening and closing their hands even during conversation and it detracts the listener greatly from the spoken words. I always thought that this was a strange behavior, a psychosomatic imbalance somewhere, until I studied Roman behavior where this was mentioned several times. Romans used copper kettles for cooking utensils and intoxicated themselves with it. When they bathed in sulfur springs, they felt the results at once. Since sulfur neutralizes the copper to some extent, it stands to reason that these people felt so very inclined to build baths even in countries outside their own, wherever a sulfur spring showed up.

Zinc is an antidote to copper. Copper easily settles in the brain and the ovaries in women. Dr. Pfeiffer made extensive studies on this subject. His book is called *Mental and Elemental Nutrients*. Please read it.

It is known that arsenic poison is likely to settle in the muscles of the back. Its presence easily contracts the muscles and the tortured muscles go into spasms and pull the spine out of place. Yellow dock and bugleweed, in equal parts made to a tea, is an antidote to arsenic poisoning.

The iron of yellow dock and tannic acid of bugleweed pick up arsenic by forming iron arsenic which the body can eliminate very early.

Another recipe is:

    grassia
    white oak bark
    goldenrod

Equal parts. Drink two cups daily.

B. Nickel

One of my sons, when thirteen, started to complain about severe backache. He was listless and complained of a stuffed up nose. Later, headaches tortured him daily. When fourteen, he slumped over the table unable to finish his homework. Instead of playing, he lay on the floor. Every morning I found his pillow wet from tears he shed from pain and despair. We had done everything. Our meager income went to physicians, chiropractors and osteopaths. Four weeks in a famous Marquet, Michigan, clinic brought no light. Two weeks at Ann Arbor brought no help. By age fifteen he was paralyzed and we had to accept it. No one can understand the suffering we parents went through.

Just to help him to get his severe sinuses opened, I started to steam poppy seed and poppy flowers and let him inhale it. It is an old German recipe which I remembered. It did him so much good and the boy, now fifteen, had such a craving for the tea that he drank several cups of it. That night he slept well and the next morning his sinuses seemed better. We did this every evening. We steamed his face with poppy seed and flowers and I boiled poppy seed for him to drink. In less than fourteen days, his pain in the back started to leave and, two months later, he was up and around, getting his strength back by swimming and exercise.

Years passed. I forgot the incident. When I stumbled over the research of biochemist C. Edgar Adelheim and the findings of Dr. Stehr, I remembered and I have to give these findings to you. It may be the answer to your problem. Dr. Stehr found that too much nickel entering the human body may paralyze the spinal column. It may bring an overflow of blood to the brain and can even bring on epilepsy. He found that the antidote is antimonial wine or opium. Poppy seed has a tiny amount of opium. When given poppy seeds, nickel deposits disappear in two months without any side effects. Poppy seeds are harmless.

When all efforts are made to correct your sinus condition, why not try the delicious poppy seeds? When everything fails to relieve the swollen knee and ankle, the painful cracking neck, stuff some

36

poppy seeds in a woman's stocking and apply to the area. When the pain is relieved in due time, praise the Lord and take a tablespoon of poppy seeds with honey by mouth twice a day or eat delicious poppy seed cake.

Research found that every second or third person has some kind of nickel poisoning. Great effort is made in England to eliminate every nickel compound from food. But, since we have nothing else as a catalyst, we have to use nickel to make hardened fats. We as homemakers can help ourselves to eliminate the danger by eating poppy seeds, poppy seed cake and rolls with poppy seeds which are delicious.

Mrs. Right was in a wheelchair. Great pain while moving tortured her. The right knee was swollen and her wrists were out of shape, stiff and painful. She had been on many cleansing programs, diets, aspirin and cortisone but nothing really relieved the pain. "If it would not be so painful at night," she sobbed. The nights were more painful than the days and sleeplessness brought her down to a twenty pound underweight condition. When she heard about poppy seed, her sister had to take off her stockings and fill them with seeds. "It feels so soothing," she said. No one could take her poppy seed decoration from wrist or knee. The night was a lot easier and, when she also took poppy seeds by mouth, the swelling and the pain left. After several weeks the wheelchair was pushed aside and, later on, sold to another unhappy sufferer.

The lowly poppy seed is the antidote to nickel. Soak one tablespoon poppy seed in juice or water. Let sit overnight and drink it the next morning. Soak another tablespoon in juice or water and drink it in the evening.

Biochemist Adelheim gave the following short extraction as a contribution to my book:

HOW THE ELEMENT **NICKEL** ENTERS THE HUMAN BODY THROUGH USAGE OF FOODS CONTAINING HYDROGENATED (synonymous with "hardened vegetable oil" being used on labels to confuse the consumer!) OILS, INDICATED ON THE LABELS OF CERTAIN FOODS, COMMONLY EATEN, **IN FINE PRINT:**

Van Nostrand's Scientific Encyclopedia, 4th Edition, 1968. p. 1186: Nickel "Finely divided nickel dissolves 17 times its own volume of hydrogen, and is extensively used as a catalyzer in the hydrogenation of oils."

pp. 870-1: Hydrogenation "Nickel, prepared in finely divided form by reduction of nickel oxide in a stream of hydrogen gas at about 300°C, was introduced by Sabatier (1897) as a catalyst for the reaction of hydrogen with unsaturated organic substances to be conducted at about 175°C. Nickel has proved to be one of the most successful in such reactions. Unsaturated organic substances containing double and/or triple bonds may be hydrogenated.

International Encyclopedia of Chemical Science, D. Van Nostrand, 1964. p. 567: "Hydrogenation increases the heat content (caloric value) of an unsaturated compound when converted into the corresponding saturated compound with gaseous hydrogen."

There is one more thing to say. Do not forget homeopathy! Like attracts like. The vibration of arsenic will pull out arsenic, will neutralize arsenic. As goes for them all.

It is in your hands to find the things needed. A psychic puts out a machine which neutralizes heavy metals and toxins in your food. Another person puts out a light which will do the same. The pressure of despair brings to us new inventions. You are not lost. Help is around you but you must seek it out.

"God helps those who help themselves."

Not your government, nor your physician but you, and you alone, will be able to protect your beloved ones and yourself.

C. Heavy Metal Reference

Poisons	Symptoms	Antidote
Gold	Tingling through system	Sulfur
Platinum	Numbness in spine and extremities	Sulfur and cold water
Silver	Cold numbness through heart region; heavy weight on hands and feet	Barley water
Lead	Exhaustion; in children hyperactivity	See recipes in book; Plumbum
Mercury	Hyperactivity	Warmth and sulfur baths
Copper	Burning sensation in throat and tonsils and through system; wants to open hands all the time	Zinc plus B_6; Sulfur baths; Cuprum
Arsenic	Hot burning sensation in the eyes, throat and chest; enlargement of tonsils	Sulfur; See herbal recipes; Arsenicum
Tin	Cold, icy feeling throughout body; numbness of feet	Salt placed in hands
Bismuth	Sensation of fullness of blood and congestion of arteries	Metallic tin placed in hands
Nickel	Overflow of blood to brain; paralysis of spinal column; epilepsy	Magnesia in both hands or internally; Poppy seeds
Graphite	Sense of numbness all over body	Poppy seed recipe
Cobalt	Disposition to hemorrhage	Oysters eaten uncooked; Bathe hands and feet in cold water; Sodium bicarbonate

These findings are from Dr. Stehr, M.D.

Magnetism

Science teaches us that different bodies can occupy the same space if these bodies are on a different vibrational level. For example, our surrounding atmosphere is filled with light waves, sound waves, heat waves, odic force, electricity, magnetism, gases, water vapor and many unsolved mysteries. But all these do not collide, explode or interfere with each other because they operate on different vibrational levels and rates. You know that many calls can be made through one telephone line at the same time because each call is sent on a different vibrational rate.

The same is true in the human body. As far as we know now, we have five bodies. They occupy the same space but vibrate on different levels. There is the physical body. It is the body we see and feel, the body which hurts when we pinch it, the body whose bones can break and whose skin can be injured by pressure or knife. The medical physician is well trained to take care of this body.

Another body is the mental body. It cannot be seen, felt or cut with a knife, bent, broken, beaten up or stamped on but it occupies the same space as the physical body and psychiatrists are trained to help when this mental body needs help.

Churches preoccupy themselves with the understanding and teaching of the spiritual body and chiropractors are trained to take care of the coarse electromotive body of the human machine. The coarse electromotive body runs through the nervous system and has its stem in the spinal column. By keeping this spinal column and other nerve paths in good health, the chiropractor helps his patients to achieve good electromotivation of the finer body, therefore, better circulation of the physical body.

There is one more force occupying the same space as our physical body. This has no name as yet, so we call it "Gauss magnetics." It is of finer electromotive vibration and it has its seat in the lymphatic system of our body. There, in the lymphatics, it can be contacted by pressure or with the Chinese method of acupuncture. This finest of the five bodies, as we know it now, bridges the gap between the physical, as our allopathic doctors know, and the spiritual, as the churches teach and know about. It is the body which carries universal electric force through our system and we all know that, without these universal high vibrational forces, there would be no life possible.

The Gauss magnetics is a body which contacts every cell and every nerve in our body. It is the true blueprint after which life form takes place. Through the finest, intangible channels, the power of the universe has its being. The universal force enters through the left hand, passes by will through the right hand and involuntarily through the right foot back to the earth and universe. That means we can direct the universal force by will through our right hand to heal and soothe and balance conditions that are out of order. If we do not exercise will, the force flows through us and leaves the body through the right foot.

Up to now the existence of Gauss magnetics was denied because no channel has ever been found on a cadaver. Postmortems do not show any such channels. The reason for this is that the lymphatic system and the channels collapse at once at death. However, there are twenty chains known and any stoppage in one of these chains may result in physical or mental difficulties. Gauss magnetics has been known to the Chinese people for centuries. They call it acupuncture. Acupuncture, as the Chinese teach and use it, is designed to open blocked channels in this finest of our bodies. There is no doubt that, with intense studies, feeling and intuition, these people have developed a healing system par excellence which works for the Eastern races. Unfortunately, the puncturing of the skin with different needles, gold, silver and others, to different depths of the tissue does not have the same desired quick healing result in people of the Western hemisphere. I often wondered why and asked and observed until one Japanese physician told me that the Westerners have a slightly different physiological makeup and the finer bodies cannot be reached by acupuncture in the same satisfactory way as in the Easterner. That means we have to get busy and find our own way to contact the channels of Gauss magnetics.

The Bible talks about contact healing in several passages and I often wondered what this is all about. I felt that there was a deep understanding and a deeper meaning in these passages and it had to do with the "laying on of hands." However, when the laying on of hands is done in a scientific manner by knowing the passages of Gauss magnetics, by contacting important points of this system, the laying on of hands becomes an art of grace and knowledge. Every physician can use the old-time method of the Bible to the greatest benefit of his clientele.

I am eternally grateful to God for bringing me in contact with an American physician who, through divine guidance, found the keyboard to Gauss magnetics (contact healing) for us Westerners. His name is Rev. Dr. Francis M. Houston, who developed a scientific method to open the finest of our bodies through contact by hand and fingertip. When the channels of Gauss magnetics are blocked, stopped up, reversed or otherwise not functioning, contact healing comes to the rescue. It is the Western way of acupuncture. As acupuncture brings reliable results to Chinese and Japanese people when Gauss magnetics is involved, contact healing brings reliable results to us Westerners when Gauss magnetics needs help.

The helping hand you always looked for is on your own arm. You have a mind to direct the hand. God gave you your mind to study. Why don't you take up the tremendous knowledge of contact healing as given by one of our greatest living brothers, Rev. Dr. Francis M. Houston of Pine Valley, California.

Magnetism, as used in healing, had been known throughout the dark ages and, before that, every civilization gap went back to the use of magnetism for healing. By magnetism I do not mean hypnosis. These are two entirely different subjects. Hypnosis is the use of mind matter for one particular task. For example, there is self-hypnosis. You tell yourself one word or sentence or idea over and over until you believe it and it becomes a part of yourself. Or someone else hypnotizes you. He puts his mind force over your mind force like a darkening cloud and you cannot establish your own pattern of thought. Like all forces, it can be used for good or bad, constructive or destructive, healing or destroying.

Magnetism is, scientifically speaking, the mitogenic power, the mitogenic rays of the human body. These rays are found to be created between the frontal lobes of the brain. When the frontal lobes are closer together, more of the mitogenic rays are released. Quantity and quality depend and change with the polarities of the body. Magnetism is not electricity, even so it acts similarly. It is, as one schools states, an offshoot of electricity released by the body.

In the East, the magnetic energy is called the Astral Fire. If one has a sufficient amount of Astral Fire, he is vital, alive with attractive personality and he attracts things to him because magnetic quantity will attract greater quantities.

Now pause and, in your thoughts, go to visit your partners, your friends and yourself. Here is the secretary—vivacious, happy, of utmost efficiency, kind and considerate. Her activity is contagious, her smile genuine, her work is done like a breeze in sunshine. Next in your acquaintances is the listless man—always tired, neurotic, nagging, never happy, without glow and shine. Another of your friends is the old couple—always ready to help and comfort, early mornings they take a walk or tend the garden, neighbors pause to chat and receive their magnetism and grace with a bunch of flowers or a basket of fruit. And here is Nelly—the woman who only talks of her illnesses and failures along the road, she sees the thistles in her garden but not the flowers and, strangely enough, all sorts of mishaps are following her path of life.

Coming back to the manifestation of this magnetic energy in our body, we understand that the mitogenic rays are formed between the two frontal lobes of the brain. The quantity can even be measured. Some people have a great deal more of magnetic power released than others. This is the reason that some have more natural healing power than others. Everyone has healing power. Every mother can soothe her child in pain, fear or agony. Every loving hand can release headaches, tenseness and disharmony.

Science neglected magnetism and concentrated solely on electricity. Magnetism, however, has immensely greater possibilities to mankind, particularly in healing the sick. Some of us have trained ourselves in long hours of work to direct and release the healing emanation through the right hand and, therefore, to have more results than others. However, the healing power is in all of us.

There is another power joining the mitogenic waves generated between the frontal lobes of the brain. This is the earth magnetism. This power and strength is free for the taking and can be used at will. It enters through the left hand, is magnified and made usable in the seat of the mitogenic wave and can be directed by will. It emanates through the right eye, the right hand, the right hip and the right foot.

At Cornell University, a discovery was made that emanation, either from the right hand or right eye, may destroy the microorganisms of yeast. They found that when those emanations are directed by the will, the time required to destroy the microorganisms is considerably reduced.

Magnetic healing is not spiritual healing. Magnetism is a power which science knows to exist. It has not been made workable as electricity which has been put to many uses. Science found out that magnetic energy is of a certain definite octave of vibration. For instance, human magnetism, the mitogenic waves, vibrates within the infrared rays and is detectable with instruments which are adjustable to the reception of this particular wavelength.

Magnetic force influences the psychometer (pendulum) and is based on the magnetic stream of the universe. In the fine optic instruments used to photograph the planets, magnetic energy is put to use. Water dousing and other arts have been practiced for centuries. We have just forgotten how to use the magnetic forces in this day and age.

45

In case of blood clotting, one well known physician uses only magnetic healing. He sits on the left side of the patient, whose legs are flexed. Never touching the body, he places his right hand over the head. His left hand is two inches away from the tailbone.

I myself have witnessed blood clots disappearing, disintegrating in less than twenty minutes. My sister was dying. A two-inch blood clot had lodged one inch in front of her heart. The clouds of death already shadowed her face and consciousness. Her family was standing around crying and in horror when I applied magnetic healing in the above described manner. To enforce our strength we lined up one behind the other, lightly touching each other. After several minutes of silence we all heard something burst. My sister let out a scream. The blood clot had traveled through the heart in small pieces and she lived.

In South America, the old Incas held the seeds they wanted to plant in their left hand and blessed it with the right. They installed magnetic powers into the seeds to influence the future crop. We bless with the right hand because we release the mitogenic waves with the right hand and install the spoken word of love in it.

Before we go into the practical application of magnetism, I have to say one word about the polarities of the body. The quantity and quality of magnetic power depend upon and change with the polarities of the body. The right side of the body is positive, the left side of the body is negative. This does not mean good or bad by any means, these are only polarities. Nothing in the universe exists without the polarities of positive and negative. The faculties of the two sides of the body are:

Right Side	Left Side
male	female
square	round and curved
blue	gold
positive	negative
physical	spiritual
cold	warm
hard	soft
aggressive	loving
perpendicular	creative

Magnetic energy also is the carrier of vibration. It is the energy which carries the thought to the various parts of the body and, furthermore, is the carrier of thought into our affairs. The magnetic energy in a healthy person can be seen as a very faint, greyish-blue radiance. Light a pair of candles and hold a black cloth in back of your hands. Place the fingertips together and slowly pull them apart. You can see little wavy streaks coming out from the fingertips against the background. This is the color of the vibration of the magnetic energy.

The magnetic energy which is in our body has the power of healing. Of course, it is not the only power there is but many people can be returned to the road to health with the use of the magnetic healing rays.

If we build a pattern of sickness in our mind, this pattern passes into the magnetic stream and is carried to different parts of the body forming congestions which we could not get otherwise. Therefore, in all schools of esoteric teaching, much stress is laid on correct thinking. The magnetic force is the carrier of thought to the different parts of the body. The cells and the glandular system are influenced by thinking through the magnetic force.

My friend's little girl, Barbara, seventeen years old, began to fail in health. Severe headaches and vomiting spells increased from day to day in frequency and her vision was blurred. "Possible brain tumor" was the physician's findings and hospitalization was scheduled. Next evening my friend called me to ask if I could stay with Barbara a few hours since she was at the end of her rope. I gladly went and found a restless, emaciated little girl pounding her head against the pillow in agony. I sent my friend to bed and pulled a chair close. By placing my left hand over the girl's forehead, I picked up the congestion and let it run out through my right hand which I lowered to the floor. With all my mind and heart I concentrated on the flow of magnetic force through my hands. In my left hand I felt a tremendous heat building up. I felt a force pulling my right hand lower and jerking it at times. I felt a tremendous uplift, as if the room was full of holiness and divine beings.

The girl calmed down. The tortured features smoothed out slowly. In a low voice I recited the Lord's Prayer and, under the impact of this tremendous vibration, she closed her eyes and deep, regular breathing showed that finally she found some rest. I held my hand in the described manner for one hour and twenty minutes. Then I reversed it. I placed my right hand over her forehead and, with the left palm up, I gathered the magnetic stream of the universe and directed it with prayer to her aching head. A steady stream of strength ran through both of us. A warmth of indescribable nature warmed and uplifted us and the greatness of God's wonder filled the house. Next morning the headache was much better and, after several days, Barbara could go back to her tasks.

Since that time I tried it on myself. When a fruit can fell on my foot, I picked up the pain with my left hand to let it run out to the right. A burn was treated the same way. A delivery man mashed his finger in my door. It was ugly looking—blue, swollen and painful. I held his injured finger in my left hand and let the magnetic flow run down my lowered right one. The pain left, the swelling went down and he continued to work.

The Western world has, as yet, only touched the surface of knowledge regarding the human magnetism. Five thousand years ago in India, a book was written by Charaka called *Aynna Veda System*. In it is not only the perfect knowledge of material function of the body but also the magnetic functioning of the body. So this is not new. All this is as old as Methuselah.

The practical use of magnetic energies, as explained, has been used as long as mankind has existed. However, in the Middle Ages this knowledge came into discredit and was connected with evil, the devil, the dark forces. The churches burned many men and women who dared to heal wounds and sicknesses in animals and men through magnetism. Knowledge of hygiene was not in existence at that time and these poor people died by the thousands or healed themselves in secret places with herbs and magnetism.

Science nowadays recognizes the unseen powers of the universe and the mysteries of magnetism can be revealed and made workable in our lives.

Mr. Wulf was in class. He was always cold. His hands felt like ice. In a warm room he wore two sweaters. Our teacher reached over and placed an eye cap over his right eye. "Just tell us what you feel," he said. Five minutes passed when Mr. Wulf took off one of his sweaters, saying nothing. In another five minutes he said, "My feet are as warm as toast. I never had them this way." We all rushed over to feel his hands and his feet. Sure enough the polarities had changed and equalized in his body to an extent that normal temperature was obvious.

In the same class was a lady sitting isolated, close to the window, which she opened off and on to release the heat, as she said. An eye patch on her left eye made her cool down in less than five minutes. She joined the crowd and was comfortable after that. In both cases the polarities had been in imbalance. One was overfunctioning on the right side, the cold side, the refrigerator side. The woman was out of balance with polarity on her left side. The simple application of an eye patch brought, in both cases, normalcy.

There is a simple way of increasing energy. This is very good if you are tired. Raise hands over head. Close your right hand, keep the left one open and raise on your toes taking a deep breath. Let down and exhale and do this three times. You can also increase your energy any minute in your day by holding the left hand out to gather the magnetic force of the universe and, with the right hand held over your head, return it to yourself like a blessing from above. Be patient and do not touch your head. You might not feel the energy building up in your left hand the very first time.

There are herbs known to have more Astral Fire than others. The plant mistletoe, for example. The ancient Druids considered mistletoe to be a holy plant and they used it for healing and many other things. They found it to contain a great amount of Astral Fire. Also, the Canadian thistle and gotu kola, the herb from India, have more Astral Fire than any other plant.

In our exhausting modes of life, all of us complain of loss of energy, loss of vitality. Speed pills, coffee, tea, cigarettes, Coca-Cola, sugar and alcohol are consumed in enormous quantities. Why? Because we all feel a lack of energy, we are exhausted and run down. Could it be that, in our city life, we lost the connection to the source of magnetism? Our forefathers walked over a live green meadow. We tramp dead asphalt. Our grandmothers tended the garden and picked live roses. We dust artificial roses in our vases. Our grandparents ate live whole grains, we eat plastic, artificial, devitalized foods. We lost our connection to the ever renewing forces of the magnetic flow.

Our Precious Youth

There is Mike, the son a minister. His grandfather was a minister, too. The overly tall boy, age twenty-one, is thin and emaciated, so weak his hands are shaking. He is bent slightly forward, his hair dangling in long blond strands, barefooted, beads hanging around his neck, the clothes unkempt, patched. We call them the far-outs, the hippies, the flower children. There is nothing flowery to them. This boy needs help in the worst way.

There is Patricia, Pat they call her. Her long skirts made from old drapery are worn-out looking, her hair is dry and straggly and those beautiful eyes are so sad, so sad. She is the daughter of a wealthy real estate man.

What happened to the boy whose father is a famous surgeon? Listlessly, he sits in college carelessly dressed, the hair made up in a ponytail. He does not care what the professor tells the class. His thoughts are scattered, his concentration span is but half a minute long. He starts a sentence with one idea just to finish it up with the opposite statement.

What ties them together? One thing they have in common. Their hands are cold and chilly. They all have spells of great depression. They have no strength, no endurance. A great restlessness makes them travel from place to place, from state to state. The mental restlessness and inability to concentrate makes them prey to many mental and spiritual influences, teachings and dogmas. Good or bad—most of them have lost the power to decide what is good or bad for them. In short, what makes them this way? Why is the prime of our nation in such a mess? Why are they so ill, so freaked out, so tired, so disturbed, so cold and depressed?

I have spoken to many, seeking to understand them, to understand their sorrow. One of them told me, "The only time we feel halfway decent is when we take pot (marihuana)." "Boy," I answered, "you are twenty-one years old, aren't you feeling young and buoyant and strong and happy as we did when we were that age?" He shook his head. "No, Hanna," he said. "I don't. I feel cold and uncertain. I belong to no one. I feel cheated, depressed to the point of suicide. I am hungry but cannot eat. I am tired but cannot sleep. I cannot think anymore. I do not know what to do." Another said, "We do not belong to society any more. We do not belong to any church since we found that God is in the inner and not in the outer. We have no church or minister that will understand. The imminent experience of God in opposition to the transcendental God experience of the orthodox churches make the gap between old and young."

I sat down when Nil told me this. My head was twirling, my heart was aching. I knew he was right. My own girl, nineteen, was in the same condition. Cold, freaky, not able to think, chills, restless, sleepless, mentally disturbed. "God, oh God," I said, "here is something I have to find." I searched, I prayed, I worked and asked question after question. I spent hundreds of dollars on vitamins and food to help these children and my own daughter. Nothing happened. Then I met Binky. A beautiful young lady, the silent leader of a commune of twenty people. The purity of her heart radiated wherever she was. She worked for long hours as if there would be no tomorrow. Exhausted, she leaned back in her chair. The cheeks flushed, hands like ice, her thoughts far-out, she told me of her spiritual drive, her closeness to the indwelling God, her experiences in metaphysics and I knew every word was true, pure and beautiful. There was no falsehood in this flower child.

But the restlessness grew in her from day to day until she asked me to release her from work just to go to California. "I will be back," she said and waved her small hands in the doorway. She never returned. The car she was riding in with five others overturned and four youngsters were dead.

It was but two weeks after her death that I had the vision how to help these kids. Was it Binky who helped from the other side? I will never know. I prayed before my beloved Christ picture and asked for help. I had the feeling that my prayer was answered. Coming back to my desk I saw clearly written the word "basil" on a white sheet of paper. It vanished before my eyes. I knew that I had been answered. The hours to dawn were so long. Finally, at 7 a.m., I called a doctor friend in a laboratory to check this herb out. It was but fifteen minutes later when I had the answer. Sweet basil will make the difference in my child.

It not only made the difference in my young girl, many boys and girls are taking it with best results. The sleeplessness is the first to disappear, the appetite comes back, the chills and coldness vanishes, the restlessness disappears and, by and by, as the weeks pass the depression leaves.

My inquisitive mind drove me from physician to physician, from biochemist to biochemist, and this is what I was told: Polio is conquered, however, the weakened virus hypersynthesized (married) with a flu virus to form a creation, a new virus, which makes the youth so ill. I am not a chemist or a biochemist. I just write it down in plain language what I was told and, please scientists, chemists, help to find the truth about this.

Recipe given through prayer: Grind basil to powder, take one level teaspoon three times daily or stuff it in a capsule. Take it six to eight weeks or longer. Take plenty of good nourishing foods, too.

I am convinced that the youth who experience the insanity of the above illness, who go through hell fire of depression and are cast out by society, will, when returned to sanity and health, offer something to mankind that will uplift our nation to spiritual experiences of greatest dimensions.

We blame our youth for taking marihuana. As I compile the reports from all the people I talked to, and there are many, many,

53

and the terrible experience I had with my own daughter over the years, I surely cannot blame anyone for taking pot. When they smoke it, the chilliness leaves. For a little while their thinking becomes clearer. They feel at home with themselves and not in the schizophrenic condition of separation. They fall into a natural sleep which their illness does not permit them to have. I experienced all this first hand. For years I slept holding my daughter in my arms, trying to conquer her chills, her restlessness, her sleeplessness, the insanity of her dreams and wakefulness, her terrible fears to be left alone. I took her from physician to physician. Since this illness is so new, no one could give me the answer. Maybe marihuana would have helped her—it smells like basil.

In any case, I am not for marihuana but I cannot blame anyone that takes it because it **was** the only refuge the youth has had in the time past.

The use of marihuana easily leads to LSD. Please, my dear friends, don't take that! Yes, it gives hallucinations and experiences that no other drug will give but it also tears your astral body and the holy chakras to pieces. The throat center is the first to go. The heart center and the pituitary centers are next. You invite so much trouble for the coming years and your future. You simply cannot afford to take LSD in any form. There are not enough trained people and ministers to close your astral body once it is opened and damaged and I know of no herb to do so. Chaparral will take the residue of LSD out of your system. So once you decide to quit that devil stuff, take chaparral so you will have no recurrences of hallucinations. Chaparral is an herb from the desert. It cleanses the liver when taken in small doses for three weeks. Six tablets of chaparral a day for a period of ten days cleans out LSD residue. This is one of many reports.

Two lovely youngsters had taken LSD for some time. Karin, a physician's daughter form New York, was carelessly dressed. She had lost fifteen pounds and looked sick and run-down. She had dropped all classes but two and had trouble in keeping those up.

Eric was pale and somewhat shaky. He had dropped out of last semester to make money, he said, but he could not keep a job.

I sent them to Wardenburg medical center at the campus but no illness could be found. When they came back, I asked them to take chaparral tablets in order to counteract the LSD they had taken. I also asked them to write down what they experienced in the following ten days. Here is their report:

Eric

1st Day: Sorry to take those creosote smelling tablets but I promised.

2nd Day: I wonder if Karin takes them?

3rd Day: My head feels so light, I did not realize there was a pressure.

4th Day: All day I was angry at the world. I smeared the mirror full of shaving cream. I am furious and cannot stand myself.

5th Day: I feel relaxed, relaxed. I can sleep.

6th Day: I have yet to meet Karin and arrange for a date.

7th Day: I can see better. I feel free and strong. I can think.

10th Day: What a stupid fool I was to drop last semester.

Karin

1st Day: I have to hold my nose to down these evil smelling pills.

2nd Day: The constant pressure from my head left me.

3rd Day: I cried and cried all day.

4th Day: I wrote a long letter to my parents. My parents are wonderful.

5th Day: I called my parents. I feel so free.

6th Day: I took a good look at myself in the mirror. I look awful. I have to get me a dress that fits.

7th Day: I saw Eric! What a change in him. Oh God, how wonderful!

10th Day: Father is coming. We all will go and see Hanna.

They came. What a change! What lovely people God created. Thanks goes to Him!

Metabolic Diseases and Enzymes

We are inclined to think that diseases of the metabolism and changes in cell structure and so on are appearances of this day and age only. This is not so. Reports are manifold that our forefathers, and also previous civilizations, had gout, arthritis, lumbago, diabetes and tumors as we do now.

There is a reason that, in our time, these diseases are more prevalent. In fact, the increase in metabolic disharmony and illness is now out of proportion and there is no hope for immediate relief of this situation. I say immediate relief because our outstanding scientists and biochemists pointed out a way which we can walk safely.

We do not have to be afraid of old age suffering coming to us at an age of twenty-five. Arthritis, diabetes, rheumatism, lumbago and all the many diseases going under the list of metabolic diseases do not have to be a fear monster living around the corner of next year. It is freely accepted in society that one suffers from arthritis at thirty-five or forty and hyperinsulinism and hay fever become the fashion diseases of the folks in their twenties and thirties.

What did our forefathers do and eat differently that made them stronger than we are? I own a cookbook with recipes from my grandmother and great-grandmother. Part of the recipes are handwritten. One recipe for sauerkraut calls for ham and one-half pound of butter added for six people only and so on and so on. I should say that our cookbooks are more careful in suggesting heavy foods, very much to the benefit of liver, pancreas, waistline and heart. So it could not be that their cooking was more healthful when I judge from these formidable recipes. However, these people had nonchemical foods, homegrown vegetables, fertile eggs and barnyard chickens and roosters. They had corn fed beef and raw milk and cream. With these things they started to cook and, unfortunately, they cooked plenty rich.

A. Enzymes: The Miracle Workers

Up to now we have had no scientific knowledge whatsoever as to why some foods are better than others. Our forefathers ate what they liked without much consideration to cholesterol, arthritis or gout. But their natural food preserved the natural instinct of taste and this is what guided them over severe problems. If they were sick, they did not eat but just had well water and herbal teas. If they overate, they skipped a meal or two (there were no Rolaids at that time). If the children were feverish, fruit juice and water was their fare. I remember that I had to eat strongly toasted flour cooked in water for severe dysentery for a whole week and there was no salt, butter or sugar in it either. Our forefathers' instincts were keen and, with this instinct, they picked their food as they saw fit.

This instinct is lost. The refinement and chemicalization of our time has dulled our taste and we no longer can choose by taste alone. However, our rescue is close. Prominent people like Professor Otto Warburg and Professor Linus Pauling, both awarded with the Nobel prize, physicians like Holger Metz and Professor Brauchle, nutritionists like Dr. Carlton Fredericks and Dr. Carlton Wade, our beloved Mrs. Adelle Davis and wonderful Linda Clark and Catherine Ellwood all help us to get well and to stay well through scientific knowledge. Back breaking and expensive research was done for us so we can eat scientifically. The preparation of foods has been emancipated from the art of cooking to a terrifically interesting science project.

I take the privilege of summing up the many scientific reports on my desk and bringing them to a workable, happy medium and understanding for us homemakers.

We need minerals. I am speaking of inorganic minerals which the body needs as a catalyst for the different processes. For example, we need iron and copper as a catalytic agent to pick up oxygen and carry it through the bloodstream. We need inorganic calcium and magnesium. We need gold and the so-called trace minerals. All these inorganic minerals are workers in our body to fulfill the different metabolic processes which life is about. However, when it comes to the building of enzymes, inorganic minerals will not do. Now, what are enzymes? Enzymes are agents of life. No biochemical process takes place without enzymes. In order that these highly needed enzymes can be formed, two ingredients have to be present. The first one is organic minerals and the second one is raw protein. The protein factor is called the "apoferment" and the organic, mineral-loaded co-enzyme is called "coferment" (Dr. Holger Metz). In other words, organic minerals and raw proteins are biocatalysts and are needed so the body can make its own enzymes.

Now we think we have it made by eating lots of well-done meat and drinking mineral water. Unfortunately, it is not that easy. Hundreds of scientific test showed that cooked meat, hard- or soft-boiled eggs, deep frozen chicken, deep frozen protein and soy products are used by the body to build muscle tissue, bone structure, hair, skin tissue and so on; but when it comes to forming enzymes, this kind of protein will not do. It must be a raw protein and it must be unheated, unfrozen and nonchemical. When any acid, alkali or chemical is added, the protein is changed and rendered unfit for the production of enzyme. Here is where we have to use our heads. Every day we have to eat, besides protein and inorganic minerals, some organic minerals and raw protein so enzymes can be formed properly. Here is the prevention of disease. It is here that we have to change our diet. Chemicals in food will destroy precious raw protein, so will heating and freezing. Mineral poor plants will not supply our need for organic minerals.

Diseases of the metabolism are, as all scientists agree, the inability of the body to make the right kind of enzyme or to make a sufficient amount of such. Now we homemakers can help. Thank God He made scientists that not only take interest in interplanetary travels but also take interest in how we can have healthy families. Since it is proven that enzymes are the real agents of life, we homemakers have to provide the building stones for it. Besides cooked proteins, we have to make provisions for serving raw proteins as well. There are sprouted grains and sprouted seeds which have raw proteins as well as organic minerals. Raw milk, clabbered milk, finely grated raw almonds and rice polishings are loaded with raw proteins, organic minerals and B vitamins.

Brewer's yeast, preferably in the liquid state, is an excellent source of raw protein.

Organic minerals are spiritualized inorganic minerals. Organic minerals have to be induced through organically grown vegetables and fruits without spray. I say it must be without spray because spray keeps organic minerals in a shell such that the body cannot use them for enzyme production.

B. Ten-Day Regimen to Re-Establish Proper Enzyme Functioning

one pint freshly squeezed orange juice
one pint freshly squeezed grapefruit juice
one pint water with the juice of three limes
one pint water with the juice of two lemons
one pint frozen pineapple juice, diluted
one pint papaya juice, diluted
twelve whole eggs
six egg yolks
frozen raspberries or strawberries add a delicious flavor
beat eggs and mix into fruit juice mixture

This is one day's supply. For breakfast eat one kind of fresh fruit.

For lunch eat green salad and/or sprouts with raw almond dressing.

For supper eat green salad and/or sprouts with almond dressing and one steamed vegetable.

The Kidneys

The Druids considered the kidneys of animals sacred and these were not eaten but buried under large oak trees. The bean shaped organ must have impressed these people or perhaps they had an inner knowing about these valuable organs. In any case, these old-timers had respect for kidneys and their functions and every year they secured a large variety of herbs by drying and storing them for winter use. These herbs were shave grass and chamomile. Birch leaves and white nettle were dried, too, and, in the fall, they gathered rosehips.

In the Middle Ages shave grass was used most widely and, in old writings, stories and descriptions of herbs kept secretly in monasteries, shave grass was number one used for kidney troubles.

I found something very interesting about what these people did. They stuffed the mattresses of kidney sufferers with either male or female fern. I found a detailed description when to use male fern and when to use female fern. Male fern was used when the right kidney was not functioning, female fern was used when the left kidney was not functioning.

In later works on herbology of the Middle Ages (about 1806), the distinction of female and male fern was dropped and it was advised to sleep on ferns.

We all know that our kidneys are filters. When the kidney quits its job, we certainly are in for troubles. The waste and the water is not carried away and it builds up, fills the subcutaneous tissue and, by and by, hinders the normal functioning of the human body. Dr. Alexis Carrel showed with the experiment of the chicken heart that, for life purposes, it is just as vital to feed the right nutrition as to carry away the waste material and this is just what the kidney filters are designed for.

Going back to our old-timers, who made a separation of male and female remedies for the kidneys, I stumbled onto a paper of a most modern scientist, a man whose knowledge and findings will be recognized forty to sixty years from now. He is a man whose foresight is so tremendous that I sit in awe and greatest admiration at his feet to listen to every word of wisdom. Unfortunately, he wants to be unnamed, unmentioned and I respect him too much to offend his wishes in any way. This man told me that the right kidney takes care of the waste below the middle of the body which is yang in nature and the left kidney takes care of the waste material of the upper part of the body. The difficulties in the proper remedies pertaining to kidney dysfunction seem to be our misunderstanding of the proper functioning of such.

So we actually need two remedies—one for the malfunctioning of the right kidney and one for the malfunctioning of the left kidney. Here comes the knowledge of our old-timers. In some cases they took female ferns and related herbs and stuffed them in their bedsteads and in other cases they used male fern. How they found out which kidney was at fault without our shining laboratories, our test tubes, our expensive outfits, is to me a riddle. In admiration I dig in these old books to compile this new modern version of old-time remedies and with it I stumble over the most recent discoveries which will shake an old belief of kidney malfunctioning.

It is a fact that men suffer a great deal more from kidney ailments of the right kidney and women more from ailments of the left kidney. It is peculiar that it is so and no extra thought was ever put on the frequency of this phenomenon. While studying the works of a famous herbologist, I found that for restoring the functions of the right kidney the following herbs are particularly beneficial: pumpkin seed tea, watermelon seed tea, shave grass tea and male fern tea. For the left kidney: cornsilk, uva ursi, fresh watermelon and female fern are more in order.

When both kidneys are impaired in their functioning, chamomile tea should be taken and should be continued to be taken a month after all signs of illness are gone.

A lady from Nebraska sent me the following recipe. It was handed down from generation to generation. She was so kind to share with me this most effective, most valuable recipe which everyone can do in their own kitchen. Take one handful of unsprayed potato peelings and cover them with two cups water. Simmer (low heat) for fifteen minutes and strain. Take two tablespoons of this potato concoction in one glass of water and drink four glasses a day for fourteen days. After several days you will see the swollen ankles and legs regain their normal size. Try it. It cannot hurt anyone and will in no way interfere with medications of any kind.

The overworked kidney often times expresses its dire need for attention in sore and painful knees. When it becomes painful to the knee to raise your foot from step to step on a stairway, see your physician and take a urine sample to him. Also, when your eyesight is dimmer in the mornings than in the evenings or when sparks appear at odd times of the day, take your urine to a laboratory to make sure your kidney is not involved.

How did people formerly find out when the kidneys were not functioning right? They boiled one cup of the first morning's urine and added one teaspoon of vinegar. The urine would coagulate when albumin was present and our old-timers took care of it with herbs. For albumin, they took motherwort. When the urine showed blood, they took shepherd's purse or marshmallow root. This latter was also used for burning urine.

The herb uva ursi is found in forests all over the world and is an old, old remedy for bladder trouble. It was used alone or in combinations with other herbs to relieve discomfort and promote healing of the urinary tract. The first time I saw it used was in the modern clinic of Professor Brauchle. He was so successful that many modern clinics adopted his suggestion and it is widely used in gynecological sections of modern hospitals as a routine drink after operations or childbirth. With the help of this herbal tea, the time spent by nurses on catheter work was cut to one-fifth and nurses, as well as patients, were relieved from this dreaded performance. I myself had to use the tea several times. It tastes bitter, but not ugly bitter, and it should be taken hot. After the first eight ounces a marked relief of tension is noticed and, taken every two hours, burning of the bladder soon leaves. Unfortunately, I could not interest any laboratory to find out what it is that is of such great benefit. It could not be sheer suggestion. Gynecologists would not allow it in their clinics as a standard routine if it would not help to relieve discomfort, save time for nurses and promote healing.

The Stomach

Our stomach is an organ neither yin nor yang, neither positive nor negative, and has its own way of operating. There are 50,000 glands ready to dissolve, prepare, harmonize, liquefy and electrify the food we are taking in. The stomach is very emotional. One notices this particularly in children. When they are upset, they complain of stomachache. Pain and discomfort somewhere else gives them pain in the stomach. Young women have the tendency to throw up and men and women faint when seeing blood or emergencies because the stomach contracts so suddenly that it shuts off all connections for a little while. Unfortunately, our stomachs are very abused nowadays and the stomach's capacity of digesting the food we fill it with is greatly overtaxed. A cocktail stimulates the stomach glands and these industrious little workers pour the acids, pepsin, hormones and fluids into the stomach so that it is halfway filled before you sit down for dinner. And here comes a whole spectrum of mixtures— vegetables, fruit, pie, buns, steaks, ice cold water, potatoes, sour cream, butter, ice cream and boiling hot coffee. We sink back into the chair and say, "That was good, I enjoyed the dinner. I am full and satisfied." Is your stomach satisfied too? I doubt it. The poor little man in the dark is numbed and paralyzed and cannot move. The muscles of the stomach will have to give so there is room to work—a worktable so to speak. But the gases of the mixture will start occupying the room and the stomach muscles have to give some more. The ice water has paralyzed the production of pepsin. The hot coffee has numbed the nerve control. The mixtures start gassing and the owner of the stomach has to have Alka Seltzer. Isn't that the way it goes?

Our stomach is made for simple, wholesome foods, not ice water and mixtures. Fruit and vegetables are incompatible at the same meal. In the East they know the secrets of food combining and will not offer their families fruit and vegetables at the same meal. Fruits are air food and vegetables are mineral food. Just keep them apart. Apples are neutral and can combine with either one or the other.

Wrong combinations and too much of all of it makes a thick, glue like mucous in the stomach and the trouble begins. There is a wonderful recipe which I found in an old Swedish-Finnish herbal doctor book. It must be pretty old—printed in 1890, collected from folk medicine. Thirty minutes before a meal take six ounces of warm water, add one tablespoon glycerin and one teaspoon ground hops. Hops happen to be full of natural pepsin. I converted this recipe. I bought liquid pepsin and here is the modern version of this formula. Taken long enough, it works and brings new life into the worn-out stomach.

        six ounces warm water
        one tablespoon glycerin
        one-half teaspoon pepsin
        thirty minutes before each meal

As I said, the stomach is very emotional. Old folks and our best nutritionists all say do not eat when you are upset, angry or full of hate. Your stomach is so emotional, he is crying for peace, understanding and harmony. When you fill the stomach while you are full of hate, the stomach will not produce any digestive juices and the food sits there and rots.

68

When you scold a child while he eats, immediately the stomach folds up its production of juices. Here you have the first onset of an ulcer. Love your child and his tender stomach nerves. The disciplinary words can be said much later. One of my dearest friends in New York had a very sensitive, beautiful and intuitive boy. There were some minor marriage problems, however, and the parents were unable to come to an agreement about disciplinary procedures. One day the boy smashed a window. It was on a Friday. Bob wanted to confess it right away to his father but the mother said, "Please do not do it now, your father promised to take me out and he will be so angry it will spoil my evening." That evening Bob could not eat but was forced to empty his plate. That night he was almost sleepless. In the morning he dozed off and he wet the bed. The father was already gone when Bob came to breakfast. Again he felt guilty—this time for wetting the bed. He could not eat so he drank ice cold pop and waited for the evening to tell his father about the broken window, for which he knew he would get a severe spanking, which he did.

The child grew up. Many trips to the psychiatrist were made. Stomach ulcers developed early in life and he has to eat carefully selected diets. Instead of a healthy, robust boy, we have a timid hypochondriac.

The children are coming from school. They have had an active day. The last stretch of the road after the bus left them out they were dashing and running and excited. The first trip they make is to the refrigerator to fetch a glass of ice cold milk or ice cold juice. How wonderfully it quenches the thirst, how exciting it tastes. It rolls down so smooth and easy. Down there where it is dark, it is not so easy. The coldness contracts every one of the glands. The juices of the stomach, being acid in nature, are quickly neutralized by the alkalinity of the milk and the cold cheese sits in those emotional children until very late. You wonder why Rose is so nervous, why Tim is so uneven in behavior and why little blond Marge sits over her homework and cries. She is tired and emotionally wounded. She feels sick all over her whole little body. No wonder, the coldness in an overheated body gave a jerk to the whole nervous system. Some people are more robust than others and can take more of this punishment but many, many break down early in life emotionally, nerve wise and with the host of stomach disorders medical books are full of.

Dr. Albert Schweitzer, the famous physician from the jungles of Africa, refused during his visits to America all ice water and asked for tepid water. A journalist noticed this and asked him why he was so persistent in his refusal of ice water. In his tactful way, Dr. Schweitzer explained that, if he would permit ice water to be given in his clinic, his coworkers would break down in less than two months. The tremendous impact of the temperature change would be such a jerk and jolt to the nervous system that the burden of jungle heat and African life could not be endured.

We know that glass breaks under temperature changes, that horn (handles of silverware) cannot stand hot and cold, and still we allow ourselves ice cold water, juices and milk to torture our nerves to the point of breakdown. Once stomach ulcers are established, your physician will tell you it comes from nerves, that pressure has built up, and now at last you listen and don't drink ice cold beverages any longer. Stomach ulcers can be deep and make little pain. The flat sores will give you heck. The deep ones are more serious, of course.

It is known that vitamin E heals without scars. The scars in a stomach are particularly unwanted because, in the folds of the scars, new ulcers are ready to come up.

There is a marvelous healing plant on the market. It is aloe vera. It comes in juice form. Two tablespoons in a little water several times a day takes away the pain while healing and neutralizing the overly acidic condition. It calms the 50,000 glands and makes them work more appropriately.

Stomach ulcer patients are not very cooperative and physicians can tell you story after story about that. They are emotional, easily hurt, feel insecure, sarcastic and do what they please. Therefore, herbal teas that will strengthen the nerves are very good. Old folks know this and in Europe the following formula is given by physicians:

70

two tablespoons comfrey root
two tablespoons burdock root in one quart water
boil for five minutes
drink four ounces three times daily with meals

In Japan this formula is used:

grind one cup bean sprouts
add one-half teaspoon marshmallow root
pinch of ginseng root
one teaspoon charcoal

From South America comes the following formula:

one ounce damiana leaves
one ounce chamomile
one ounce fennel
one ounce anise
boil in two quarts water for fifteen minutes
drink one cup several times a day

These herbal formulas all approach the nerve-emotional part of the picture of a stomach ulcer and have nothing to do with healing in itself, while aloe vera, bioflavonoids, vitamin E and flax seed have to do with the physical healing.

There is a little booklet on the market called *Herbal Cures of Duodenal Ulcer and Gallstones*, by Frank Roberts. It is an English publication and available at your health food stores. It is worth reading.

The closing of the stomach outlet valve is a serious problem in infants. These little ones hopelessly throw up every feeding and grow thinner and thinner. The following recipe was given to me by an old midwife in Germany. I used it on one of my children. I gave it to neighbors and friends with best results. Bring to a boil a little bit of half milk half water and thicken this with potato starch or cornstarch. You dissolve potato starch in cold water and, while stirring the boiling milk and water, let drop in as much starch as needed to make it semi-thick. No sugar. Let cool to lukewarm. From this you give one-half to one teaspoon to the infant. Wait five to six minutes and then give bottle or breast feed. The semi-thick starch mixture has relaxed the nerves to an extent that the baby can hold normal feeding. Give first a little food. Later on increase quantity. After fourteen days this extra work will not be needed and the baby can hold food without the teaspoon of starch blubber. Of course, there are always cases where an operation is needed due to other problems but just give it a try.

Trouble with the stomach often expresses itself in the neck. Many people complain about stiffness in the neck, pain in the neck, inability to turn the neck. In many cases this is a sign of lack of hydrochloric acid. Just find out what is going on in your stomach!

In order to bring and keep your active little glands in harmony, there is a wonderful help for you right at your fingertips. Have you noticed how businessmen cross their arms over their chest and hold their upper arms? I always wondered what made them do this. I also saw it when men ponder over a problem. They hold their upper arms and step back and forth in their offices, even in a lecture hall I saw this. Men do this not knowing that on the upper arm are powerful nerve reflexes leading to the stomach. While holding here they harmonize their stomach glands. The stomach sends a reflex to the brain and the brain has renewed energy. When one has stomach ulcers or trouble with the stomach, the upper arms (outside) are very sore to touch. Hold these contact points many times a day for a minute or so and in a few weeks your stomach will improve to an extent that you will enjoy a good, healthful meal without any ill effects, pains or gas (Rev. Dr. Houston).

We all have the remedy for stomach ulcers in our kitchen—the lowly potato. Juice one potato with the same amount of warm water and drink before meals three times a day. You also can grate a potato on a grater and squeeze through a cloth. It just takes a little more time and a larger potato. Later on, a piece of raw potato chewed very thoroughly before a meal feels good and relaxing to anyone that has had stomach trouble or has a weak stomach. The red potato is better for this purpose. Caution! Potato juice cannot stand at all. It has to be drunk right away.

Of course, cabbage juice is so well known for its U factor but you need a juicer and organically grown cabbage. Otherwise, the result is doubtful.

I hope I have impressed my readers to the fact that, in order to raise emotionally strong children, one has to feed the stomach to make it emotionally strong. Freshly baked breads, buns and muffins are not for tender children's stomachs. The bread should be home baked and at least one day old. Preservatives in baked goods stay preserved also in the stomach and they cannot be broken down and utilized properly.

Simple food combinations are a must to make the stomach work properly. With every meal you can change your menu. You can fix 3 x 365 dishes and menus a year. Serve only three to four things at a time but change with every meal and you have a healthy family. I call it the "Trinity Diet." For example:

Breakfast: cereal, cream and sweet fruit
or egg and toast and tea
or meat and vegetable and tea
or soup and bread

Lunch: salad and fish
or meat and one cooked vegetable
or potato and vegetable
or fruit pie and carob drink
or high protein drink and fruit

Supper: the same simplicity of one vegetable,
one protein, one salad
or potato and vegetable and salad

Remember:

1) Never eat meat and milk at the same meal.
2) Never eat fruit and vegetables at the same meal.
3) Never eat acid fruit and cereal at the same meal.

Meat and milk need two different digestive enzymes. Since Moses' time, no Hebrew serves milk and meat together and these smart people keep this rule very strictly. Fruit is cleansing, vegetable is building. Fruit is yin, vegetable is yang. When both are put together, you have a mess. It is incompatible with your electromagnetic field. Acid fruit and cereal make a glue like mixture and stick to the stomach lining and children suffer from it. Give fruit or a healthful sweet between meals (after about two hours) and your little folks will be ready for a simple meal two hours later. Fruit juice and milk are food and have to undergo digestion. When children are thirsty, give water.

I first was struck with food combining while working in the mission field. We had arranged a picnic to which we invited about three hundred peasants. We celebrated Dr. Clark's birthday and it was his desire to invite the villagers. We had salad, hot dishes, cakes, cookies and hot and cold drinks. The people filled their plates with three to four items and let their children have no more than three items on the plate. When I filled my plate with all the goodies I saw, one woman shook her head and said, "How is your stomach going to react? You will bring tears to your mother's eyes." Being seventeen, I ignored this warning. By nineteen, I had a good sized ulcer and terrible emotional upsets. I was raised on Spartan principles and I negotiated myself into illness by trying to be smarter than my parents and disregarded the simple rules of health which I saw practiced right before my eyes. Only Spartan simplicity in the choice of food brought me back to health and the little man in the dark has never bothered me since.

In Europe there are special resorts for healing stomach ulcers and this is their diet:

For the first days nothing but carrots, cooked and mashed.

On the fourth day:
Morning:	carrot soup
Mid-morning:	potato broth
Noon:	potato and carrot
Mid-afternoon:	herbal tea, cream and rice crackers
Evening:	carrots and baked potato
Bedtime:	herbal tea and cream

One week on this regimen and most people can increase their food intake to a normal, productive diet.

The Liver

The liver is one of the organs greatly afflicted in this time and age. There have been liver afflictions reported at all times. They used to call it biliousness and, when someone was listless, mentally disturbed, off his rocker, the old physicians said, "He is liverish."

The liver plays a most important role in detoxifying the bloodstream and the lymphatic system. Besides this, the liver has many other functions. The function of detoxification is greatly overtaxed. With the air, we breathe in lead from the car exhaust. With our food, we take in DDT, additives and chemicals galore. Cooking in improper cookware, we add more insult to the liver. With sprayed vegetables, we add a dash of arsenic and other no-nos—small amounts, of course, as Rachel Carson said in her book *Silent Spring*. What are we doing to counteract these poisons and help the liver? Not much. We continue our diet of fried foods, potato chips, cakes, pies and cookies until one day the liver tells us, "I have had enough," and we start feeling sick. We had been sick all the time but now we feel it. As Dr. Donsbach said, we used up all the power of the liver to detoxify and are approaching the last twenty percent of its capacity.

As I said, liver trouble was known in all ages and what did our forefathers do? There is a beautiful little story I read as a child which I have to relate to you. Once there was a very rich man whose only purpose in life seemed to be eating. He grew heavier and heavier and nastier and nastier. One day he became very ill and sent for the doctors. All the potions and pills did not help. He grew nastier and the pain grew worse. Finally, he sent to a wise man in a faraway town. This man realized that no potion would do and sent him a letter telling him, "Friend, you have a big monster in your intestine. It will eat you up. Come and see me. You have to walk all the way and eat only hard-boiled eggs and greens." The frightened man started out. He was so heavy and tired. He walked only two miles that day, cursing and aching and crying. Every day he could walk more and when, after weeks, he reached his destination, he was slim and happy and whistling and full of vim and vigor. This is one way to cure biliousness.

I have a book from the seventeenth century in which an old physician from Austria gives his secrets. One of them is the apple juice diet. This diet is greatly used among health minded people to detoxify liver and gallbladder. Here is one report. "I had a very bad summer. Too much work, too little sleep. I did not take food supplements and had to work under conditions where I had to eat fried foods and other no-no foods. In the fall it started. Tired, bloated, listless, I caught myself being sarcastic and nasty. One night I had terrible pain over my right shoulder and neck. I am sorry to say my liver quit her job and the next morning I went on the apple juice diet. The bright green pebbles, the old bile, just poured out on the third day and I was myself again."

Here it is and I recommend it to everyone very, very highly. Give your liver a rest, a chance, a holiday.

A. Apple Juice Diet

First Day

8 a.m.	one glass (eight ounces)	apple juice
10 a.m.	two glasses (sixteen ounces)	apple juice
12 p.m.	two glasses (sixteen ounces)	apple juice
2 p.m.	two glasses (sixteen ounces)	apple juice
4 p.m.	two glasses (sixteen ounces)	apple juice
6 p.m.	two glasses (sixteen ounces)	apple juice
8 p.m.	two glasses (sixteen ounces)	apple juice

Juice should be natural, without chemicals. No food is to be taken this day.

Second Day

Same procedure as the first day. No food this day either. At bedtime four ounces olive oil. You may wash the olive oil down with hot lemon juice or hot apple juice.

As a rule, this diet starts to work around 4 a.m. In the fecal matter you will find little green pebbles. They may be the size of a pinhead or they may be as big as a bird egg. Many times it all looks like green mud.

In any case, the old stagnant bile becomes dissolved and liquefied through the malic acid of the apple juice, which should be sugar and chemical free, and the oil moves the whole mess.

Dr. Adolphus Hohensee had been using this diet on thousands of his students all over America. In Europe it is practiced in health spas and hospitals with equal results. It re-establishes the normal function of the liver. This diet "frees the liver-gallbladder tract from the old bile and debris, which we call stones!!"

The old American Indian recipe for liver trouble is chaparral tea and/or fringe tree bark. Chaparral is a creosote bush from the desert and tastes very nasty. Mayo Clinic got interested in this herb and is doing research at the present time. An ingenious manufacturer made chaparral in table form and it is available in health food stores and sometimes drugstores.

All liver teas are bitter teas. It is as if nature wants to heal bitter gall with bitter teas. Dandelion leaves and root, gentian and fringe tree are relief to an ailing liver. These herbs were in use for centuries and, I am happy to say, they are still good in this day and age.

This is a recipe from South America for hepatitis. This illness is now prevalent in our far-out youth and begins to be a threat to some communities.

I knew Sheryl for some time. A lovely, fair youngster full of adventure, pep and vigor. When she left for San Francisco, she waved goodby and I had an awkward feeling. Weeks later she came back a thin, yellow youngster, scrawny hair, listless. She snatched the first chair to sit down. "Sheryl," I said, "what did you do?" Hepatitis," she said, "just dismissed from five weeks' hospital stay." Tears came to my eyes. Where was the happy youth? A suffering thin little bundle of a formerly happy Sheryl stared with big eyes into emptiness.

I told her about the old recipe of the Indians in South America and, in addition, I told her to simmer lettuce leaves (loose leafed lettuce) and spoon the water two tablespoons every hour. The week passed. Sheryl did not show up. I looked in the paper for hospital admissions daily. Nothing. Her name was not mentioned. Sunday I saw her in church. I stared at her. She was beautiful. All the yellowness was gone. A smile spread over her lovely face. Sunshine sparkled in her eyes. She seemed a lot stronger in every way and her clumsiness was gone—agile as a pussycat. Just plain lovely.

Here is the South American Indian recipe I gave Sheryl. Squeeze two to three limes, according to size, in one pint water, sweeten with one tablespoon tupelo honey or another very good raw honey. Drink as much as you can. Every time your pint is gone, make more lime water. Drink this for three days and, in addition, take two tablespoons of lettuce water every hour. No food is needed or required. On the fourth day eat beets and lightly cooked vegetables and drink more lime water. Continue adding food slowly and discontinue lime water after one week.

B. Liver Rejuvenating Recipes

I found the following recipe in an old book used in 1802 by Dr. Selig of Austria. It sounded so good that I tried it and found that it is truly excellent.

> one teaspoon dandelion root
> one teaspoon angelica or arnica
> one teaspoon wormwood
> one teaspoon gentian
> boil in two cups water, simmer and strain

Add two quarts apple juice and four ounces freshly squeezed lemon juice and drink this in small portions during the day. Do this for two to three days and repeat if needed once a month. Take only stewed fruit and apple juice on these days.

Mrs. Fisher had beautiful hands and arms but large spots of dark pigmentation covered them. These pigmentations grew worse from year to year. When I shared with her the above recipe, she was all for it—and what wonders! The dark circles and "age spots" faded and slowly disappeared.

Also for the liver: Wash one average sized grapefruit and cut in small pieces. Add one and one-half quarts water and boil for fifteen minutes. Strain off the liquid and sweeten with honey. Drink six ounces once a day (Al Wolfsun).

Everyone can afford this: Blend ten leaves of dandelion in one and one-half cups cranberry juice until liquefied. Drink in two portions. Half of it mid-mornings, the other half mid-afternoons.

Mysteriously, the liver has something to do with our cholesterol problem. We have to have some cholesterol in our body. The liver determines the size of the cholesterol molecules, the amount of such and its healthy function within a healthy body.

The Japanese contributed the following interesting research to the cholesterol problem. Dr. Hikasa was able to produce cholesterin gallstones with different diets in animals. Foods rich in glucose, with or without fats, were the ones to build cholesterin gallstones the fastest. He found that a glucose rich diet, with or without fat, accelerated the formation of cholesterin gallstones by four times. The substances he found to reduce already formed cholesterin gallstones were flax seed oil and cellulose carbohydrates, which means mainly vegetables and fruit.

The chemical picture of the formation of cholesterol stayed obscured until recently when Dr. Hikasa found that the white blood corpuscle of the blood excretes a hormone which is the building stone of lipase. Lipase is very necessary in digestion and for the proper functioning of the liver. All cholesterin high people are low in lipase, Dr. Hikasa said.

An American scientist, however, found that the hormone which is needed to form lipase is manufactured in the shinbones, the right one particularly. It is picked up by the white corpuscle and carried by it to the liver or wherever it is needed. So, the white corpuscle is only a carrier of the hormone.

Very interesting, very enlightening, very beautiful! Soon the problem of cholesterol will be licked. Meanwhile, have your liver in the best shape possible.

The Lungs

We can remain without food for four to six weeks, without water for four to six days and without air for four to six minutes. What is it that makes breathing so important? Why is it the least talked about subject? We all talk about good foods. Feasting and fasting are common subjects and books are written about the tortures of being deprived of water. But few have described the agony of not getting enough air. We should be terribly concerned about breathing but more so about the air we have to breathe.

The lung is a yin organ and is the opponent to the yang of the intestinal tract. Only because of this divinely intelligent arrangement of positive and negative, the body can live and have its being.

We all know how air is taken in through the nose and mouth into the lungs, how the gases interchange and how we exhale, leaving the oxygen for future use in our bodies. Much less known, however, is the fact that, with every breath we take in, etheric energies are taken in too. Now these etheric energies are what the yogi calls "prana" which is etheric. Prana is both positive and negative. It has two polarities and our body is made to make use of these energies. Through the right nostril we inhale positive prana, through the left nostril we inhale negative prana. Both are needed for our well being.

It is calculated that, without the influence of prana, magnetic and other forces, we could not live. We could eat day and night and starve to death on the seventh day because we could not extract enough energies from the food and drink we could take in. This is one explanation why some people can exist on very little food. Most often these are happy and balanced people and they try forever to lose weight. They have an abundance of energies and are rosy cheeked and well rounded. There are those who get so enveloped in the work they are doing (usually creative work), that they forget all about food and drink, yet they have all the energies they need to do that job. While they do their work they forget the surroundings but they do not forget to breathe and it is a balanced breathing since they are happy and balanced. More etheric energy is, therefore, extracted from the air and they experience no loss of weight or loss of energy whatsoever.

When we inhale and fill our lungs with air, the etheric energy is extracted and is drawn into the fourth dimensional tubes which lie to the right and left side of the spine. The right tube is called "Pingala" and starts on the right nostril way up in the nose. "Ida" starts on the left nostril and extends down the left side of the spine. As I said, etheric energies are positive and negative and Pingala draws the positive current while Ida draws the negative current. We are made to draw these currents alternately. One hour we draw positive and the next hour we draw negative. This is the way we are made but, when we let ourselves be disturbed emotionally, we bring this out of balance and neglect to draw the energies in the right proportions. The time we interchange from one current to the other is extremely important. These times are the creative moments of our day. In this flick of a moment our thoughts are creative. It is in this moment we experience the law of the astral universe, the law of the next dimension in which everything is formed by thought alone and in an instant.

This one flick of a moment in which we can manifest good or bad, love or hate, destruction or creation, is so important that you should never find yourself having any bad thoughts or linger on hate, destruction, death, fear, illness or divorce. You might create it right there and then. "The fear will be upon you," said the Bible. Having only good thoughts at all times, to be ready for these moments of your day, should be your concern—that the energies will manifest in good and constructiveness, in selflessness, in advancement. We have to make ourselves ready for the Lord. All the churches teach that and still they don't know that this moment comes to us every hour of our life.

We call the positive current of prana the solar energy, while the negative current is called the lunar energy. The solar energy being drawn through the right nostril is positive in nature and can be used for self-vitalization.

Place a piece of cotton in your left nostril and breathe only through the right nostril for about one hour. During that time use your thoughts. Center your thoughts upon the part of your body that needs rebuilding or rejuvenating. You will be surprised what happens.

Mary T. had a very bad cold. All the aspirins could only soothe the headache that went with it. She felt miserable all over and called for help. Besides aspirin she had nothing in the house, no linden blossom tea, no lemons for fresh juice, not even Vitamin C. Well, I told her to plug up her left nostril and to lie back to feel the healing take place. Sure enough, it took less than half an hour that Mary started to feel better and she continued to do so. She returned to work the next day.

It is known that great natural healers breathe for greater periods through the right nostril than through the left nostril. They are able to utilize and extract more solar energy than other folks can and, therefore, cannot exhaust themselves readily.

We all know of people with a very low metabolism. Mr. Hildt hardly digested his food. Everything this poor man ate literally turned to poison. Gas discomfort, sour stomach with miserable feelings after every meal, he hardly dared to sit down to the dinner table. Every day his wife turned the kitchen upside down to prepare, pulverize, grind, blend, peel and juice his food. It did not get better. Mr. Hildt got weaker and weaker. One day he got a miserable cold. His left nostril was all blocked up and he could only breathe through the right. This day his food digested well and he felt fine in his stomach. He had plenty of time to think and, when the cold disappeared toward evening, he plugged up his left nostril and started to eat. Guess what?! He experienced no discomfort. When he woke up next morning, he was hungry for the first time in a year and his head felt better. By plugging up his left nostril he balanced his polarities, the sluggish circulation stepped up and he grew better and better.

We really should make a habit of breathing through the right nostril when we eat. The solar current, the positive prana, speeds up the process of metabolism and we can digest and extract all the energy from the food we eat. We have to eat much less to be satisfied because we get so much more out of our food. On the other hand, in case you have to undergo a fast, plug up your right nostril and breathe more through the left. You will not be so hungry. It will slow down the metabolism in the body. All yogis do that in the East when they go on those long fasts and we feel so sorry for them. How tricky can you get!

Ellen was always listless, anemic, run-down, constipated and just not herself. She complained of lack of energy and dullness in her head. Treatments for anemia resulted only in temporary improvement. Everyone thought and said that she liked this condition. Her husband was a very fine person and realized that this was not the Ellen he knew. He asked for help and I suggested she plug up her left nostril so more solar energy would enter her body. This was Friday. Sunday afternoon they took a long hike to the mountains and enjoyed every moment of it. She returned refreshed and with her lovely complexion all tinted pink from the new strength and new life force. She never needed another iron pill or B_{12} injection.

Now we find individuals who have an excessively nervous temperament. Their metabolism is highly stepped up. Usually they are thin and restless and sometimes a little hard to get along with. These people would benefit greatly by breathing every day for an hour through the left nostril. The food would have time to be digested more slowly and the stepped up metabolism would become more normalized.

On the other hand, we find people who have a tendency to breathe through the left nostril too much and may have a terrific water retention and weight problem. The left breath, the Ida center, is called the moon center. To a great degree it regulates the distribution of the various fluids and secretions of the endocrine glands and the water household of the body. Since the water in our system is highly polar in nature, it stands to reason that the lunar breath has an influence on the fluidic matter in the system. These people may try to breathe through the right nostril more often to balance weight and fluid matter more thoroughly.

The techniques of breathing are discussed in many yoga lessons. Some of them are so time consuming that we Westerners with our quick actions lose patience. We do it once or twice and leave the rest to the yogi. Remember, however, when you inhale, you take in the pranic energies. Therefore, train yourself to inhale very slowly. You may exhale fast but always inhale slowly.

There are certain breaths that are used for the stimulation of the various functions of the body. We have mentioned some already. One to overcome mental lassitude and brain fatigue is very easy and can be done at any desk. Close both nostrils, inhale through the mouth and then force the breath into the nasal passages and start to exhale with the mouth closed. When this is done, the etheric current is diverted and focused into the brain cells and acts to stimulate them. Do that several times in a row and several times a day.

A. Lung Exercises

Stand or sit with the spine erect. Place the tip of the tongue at the roof of the mouth or the root of the upper row of teeth. Then close both nostrils with the fingers and inhale slowly through the mouth. Take a long deep breath until you have filled the lungs with air to full capacity. The slower you inhale the more you can take. Then slowly exhale all the breath from your lungs through the mouth. Contract the abdomen at the same time. Do that ten times. This will increase the oxygen supply in your body.

Now relax. Pucker your lips just as you do when you are going to whistle. Then close the nostrils with the fingers. Slowly inhale a deep breath through the mouth. Close the mouth and exhale slowly through the nostrils. Draw through the mouth and exhale through the nostrils ten times. This is the second exercise for the oxygenation of the bloodstream and it liberates the etheric current. The next one is very refreshing for the control of thought. Close the left nostril and inhale through the right. Count to eight while holding your breath. Preferably, take eight of your heartbeats as the amount of time. Exhale through the right nostril. Then close the right nostril and breathe through the left, count to eight while holding the breath and release through the left. Inhalation and exhalation is through the same nostril. This method will enable us to confront our problems and bring to definite and understandable conclusions that which was obscure, veiled and turmoiled. Try it.

Science declares that all things that we require for the building of our body tissues are held in suspension in the air. If this is so, every time we breathe we can draw from the atmosphere the things which are necessary for the building of our tissues, bones, nerves and all parts of the body (Dr. Doreal).

When we think of the power of breath and how important it is in our life, it sounds strange that more importance is not placed on the study of taking in life currents, energies and supplies for the body through the nostrils and the inexpensive way to attain the building stones for our bodies. Scientific breathing should be taught and practiced in every household. There is still a lot more to be accomplished with controlled breathing. I have briefly mentioned the importance of the double breath. More will be said and deeper knowledge revealed at another time.

Your demand for fresh, lead free, unpolluted air is justified. In polluted, lead laden, DDT saturated air the vital current of prana is reduced to two percent. Where are we supposed to get our energies from?

People with lung conditions are easily exhausted and tired. Besides not enough oxygen, they cannot extract enough prana from the air. Why are there sanatoriums for lung diseases in Switzerland? If it were only oxygen the incapacitated lung needed, all sanatoriums should be on the ocean. But at lower altitudes lung patients cannot extract enough prana, therefore, they feel a lot better in the pure air of Switzerland. Theories are in circulation as to why Switzerland is so healing and uplifting, stimulating and different from other parts of the mountainous world. There is but one difference—the Alps have a lot more available prana than other mountains.

Coming to specific lung ailments, there are many treatments our forefathers used and they were most successful in helping the sick. When lungs were congested, they grated onions and placed them between two layers of cloth. This poultice they applied to the front and the back of the chest and placed hot water bottles or heated stones over it.

Linden blossoms and elderberry flowers are bound to break up colds fast. You have to drink one cup every half hour until six cups are taken.

Take equal parts of pennyroyal and elderberry flowers when flu hits you.

Blessed thistle is one of the herbs used to re-establish the yin magnetic power of the lungs and is known to heal long-standing infections of the lungs.

Oatstraw, with its natural silicon, helps to strengthen the lungs. I heard of one mother who, after World War II when so may suffered from tuberculosis (TB), went out to gather the leftover stubbles in the oat fields. She boiled them and gave it to the children. None of her four children contracted TB in spite of all the contact they had with TB infected neighbors.

"All emphysema cases seem to have worms, all asthmatics build up gallstones," Professor Brauchle taught in his lectures.

The yin-yang harmony of lungs and intestine is interrupted and all effort should be made to balance the disharmony. In America, we have the wonderful aloe vera plant which the Indians used for shortness of breath. From the near East, fenugreek, the mucous solvent, is imported. Mullein leaves applied to the chest and brewed to a tea for drinking is a well known treatment and is practiced in Europe and America. In old Greece, thyme, sarsaparilla and marshmallow root were boiled in wine and sipped and the chest was rubbed with hot pepper. All herbal teas that are good for the liver seem to be bitter. All herbs that are good for the lungs seem to be mild and most of them are aromatic and very pleasant.

The tea of linden blossoms is an old-timer. In the Middle Ages the linden tree was so appreciated that it was planted in almost every town square and every little village had the center square planted with linden trees. There the young folks met in the evenings for folk dancing and chats. In daytime the young mothers met with the purpose of taking water out of the center well and the old folks sat on the benches inhaling the fragrance of these blossoms.

Linden blossoms, taken right at the beginning of a chest cold, break a cold up after the second cup. Care should be taken that you are well covered because it induces sweat and breaks the congestion by opening the pores of the skin. Compresses of linden tea are healing in old wounds and eczema. The charcoal of the linden wood has something more special yet. It neutralizes putrefaction in colon and lungs, it strengthens and heals. When there is no hope left for your patient, try the linden tree. Take one tablespoon linden charcoal in powder form, place in warm tea or soy milk and drink this amount mornings and evenings for four to six weeks. The lungs will be so strengthened that all congestion will leave in a hurry.

The pine tree was used in the Middle Ages for relief of lung congestion. Branches of pines were placed under the bed of the sufferer. The young tops of pines were placed in a vessel covered with water and simmered for two hours. After removing the twigs, the juice was boiled for another hour to make it more concentrated by evaporation. Honey was added to preserve it and it was boiled for another half hour. Placed in jars, it kept well for winter use.

Dr. Selig writes in his book *Krautergold* that the most healing are the branches of the creeping pine found high up in the mountains. Small branches are to be boiled for one hour. The brew is mixed into bath water and the patient takes a bath for fifteen minutes. Rest is indicated after that. Sickly children and people with long-standing lung congestion are so strengthened that they become healthy after only several weeks of this daily procedure.

I have seen miracles with pine concoctions concerning weakened lungs and weakened nervous systems. The sleep is deeper, breathing becomes regular and deeper after the first bath and, when you place twigs of pines under the bed and in the room, the volatile oil continues to heal all twenty-four hours long.

Whenever you see someone that cannot breathe easily, remember how lucky you are. Count your blessings. Forget the petty things that bother you and ask angelic forces to help your suffering fellow man.

Simian Virus 40

The biggest tragedy that ever hit America started in the mid-fifties. It came like a shooting star, brilliant and beautiful. It raced from coast to coast touching almost every home. Then it disappeared. But, unlike a shooting star, it left behind a trail of sorrow, despair, mental and physical illnesses, suicide, financial ruin for many families, confusion and the "hippie" problem.

It was the Salk Vaccine, the most extensive experiment on humans ever performed, and it became the biggest disaster ever known to mankind.

In the mid-fifties of this century, thousands of little rhesus apes were shipped to America. They were delivered by the truckloads to laboratories. With long needles, their little kidneys were pierced and the deathly polio virus was injected. The little animals became deathly ill, the kidney decomposing with pus and decay. On the heights of their suffering, the rhesus apes were killed and the pus extracted. This was injected into fertile eggs and, after a few days, the famous Salk Vaccine was ready to be injected into our children's bloodstreams. Many vaccines are made that way, however, here entered the tragedy. The polio virus was dead but no one knew and no one checked that, with this vaccine, a little virus had slipped in which is only known to be present in apes.

This ape virus has the scientific name of simian virus 40, in short sim 40 and sometimes SV40.

Sim 40 is harmless to apes but, when entered into the bloodstream of our children, the disaster started.

The big business, the huge propaganda machine, the praise and the advertisement subdued the cries of the parents whose children were suddenly hit with:

fear
lack of cleanliness
anguish
failing physical health
failing mental health
depression
laziness
hatred towards parents and teachers
low grade temperature
listlessness
meningitis

. . . and many more behavior symptoms which were not present before the vaccine was given. Many physicians realized very soon that something went wrong with the inoculations. To avoid more troubles for their patients, they injected sterile water until they knew what was going on and the propaganda machine became occupied with other things. It was Dr. Sabin whom God gave the wisdom, stamina and integrity to help us. Dr. Sabin also bought rhesus apes. One of his first helpers was bitten by an ape and this man developed a strange fever. It looked just like a brain fever but it was much more and carried many of the symptoms the parents noticed in their children. Dr. Sabin found sim 40 in his associate. Then he examined the Salk Vaccine and, in each vial, there was this ape virus.

Sim 40 had never been in human blood before and all at once millions of Americans had it.

Of course, many children were able to throw the virus off. But many of them, particularly the finely nerved ones, the sensitive ones, were unable to cope with it. No one understood why these children behaved so strangely. They became loners, they were chilled, cold, miserable. They became paranoid, fearful and depressed and developed suicidal tendencies. Soon they forgot to wash themselves or comb their hair, did not care about their appearance and then the parents had to throw them out of the house because it was a disgrace to see them in society.

In the streets they found company—boys and girls their age who understood what fear was. They all had the chill, they knew how terrible it was to be alone when the suicide tendency struck. They knew how the deep depression could hit and hurt.

Up in the mountain valleys they kept to themselves in flocks like sheep do. Two slept in one sleeping bag because of fear to be alone. Because of fear of the incredible nightmares, because of the chills, they went through night after night.

Many of these people are now between twenty and thirty-five years of age. Many have seen the horror of mental institutions. Many have committed suicide. Many have seen jails from the inside and many just exist.

The acute stage of this virus is over, however, it is not dead. The second episode is showing up. Many, many children, also folks between forty and sixty and senior citizens who never had the first inoculation of polio vaccine, the one which brought the tragedy, now have sim 40 in their systems. It hides in the spinal fluid, in the nervous system, and they feel tension in the backs of their necks and between their shoulder blades. According to medical textbooks, veterinarian textbooks and also research done at Colorado University, sim 40 is an RNA/DNA virus. That means it goes into the nervous system. It is the most feared of all types of viruses because it can stay dormant for many, many years just to strike whenever the system becomes low in energy.

"In less than fifteen years we fell from a healthy nation to one of the sickest nations," Bob Hoffman said in one of his lectures. And he added, "America was meeting with fifty-three nations on athletics and health and we were the last one on good health."

One clairvoyant said, "I feel death in many people, right in their necks and between the shoulders." Sim 40 may break up any day now and it is that which the Bible quotes: "When two stand in the fields, one will be taken."

Year in and year out, in despair I searched and researched every avenue open to my simple mind and understanding. I prayed for my own children, my beloved ones in the mountains and in the streets and the ones in despair all over this beautiful country. I asked for a vision to help us. He said, "My people are dying of lack of knowledge." And I believe so deeply that I asked Him for His knowledge. And Jesus Christ, in His grace, reached down to us and gave in a vision the help we need so badly. Formula:

> one-half pound basil
> one-half pound kelp
> one pound milk sugar

Grind up the herbs. Mix together. Take one teaspoon four times daily in water, juice or yogurt for at least six weeks. I have noticed that some people have a light fever for a few days. Most people feel better right away for the first time in years.

Since it is a hidden virus, it may come and go for awhile but keep on taking the formula. See your children regain their mental and physical stability. See yourself changing to better health. All who read this, please become a missionary for the Lord and for this nation's health. Pitch in, do something! No race, no creed is spared from sim 40 but the race that has been hit the hardest is the Jewish race.

Old-Time Remedies

Old-time remedies used in Europe and in America—time proven, effective, simple and different:

Gout and Stone Remedy

> one quart apple cider
> one teaspoon hydrangea root

Let these stand for twelve hours, bring to a boil, simmer. Take one-half cup three times daily.

Joints

Here is a marvelous recipe to lubricate joints and make joints supple. A young girl, a flower child, gave it to me. I wish I could show to everyone the lovely drawing she put under the recipe.

> one teaspoon turmeric
> two teaspoons almond oil
> two teaspoons soy milk powder
> one cup water
> salt and honey to taste

Heat this and serve as a lovely hot drink.

Arthritis Tortures You?

In Germany you are put on a low carbohydrate, vegetarian diet. You are sent to a resort. Psychologists try to find the resentment as causative factor for your illness. The body is massaged with castor oil and wrapped in blankets overnight. Herbal teas and compresses are administered. Special diets like Schrot diet, Waerland and Bircher Benner are used and lecithin, as well as homeopathic remedies, are widely advocated.

For arthritis the Italians mix eight ounces liquid B-complex syrup and four ounces glycerin. They take six teaspoons of this mixture a day. Diluted glycerin dissolves hardened mucous collections.

In England they take six tablets magnesium oxide and ten drops phosphorus compound to counteract calcium deposits. Magnesium oxide removes calcium deposits.

In America we follow Mrs. Adelle Davis' stress formula and Dr. Warmbrand's diet suggestion.

In Turkey they bathe in hot springs and wrap the limbs with comfrey leaves.

Dr. Vogel, M.D., a Swiss physician, writes in his book *The Nature Doctor*:
> Before breakfast drink one-half glass of raw potato juice.
> One hour before midday meal chew three juniper berries.
> After meal swallow three mustard seeds.
> Between meals drink plenty of potato water.

And cover the affected parts with healing clay or cottage cheese. The diet should be absolutely natural.

He recommends goldenrod, yarrow tincture, arnica, St. John's wort and minerals from alfalfa. He writes that butterbur and mistletoe preparation regenerates the affected area.

What did our forefathers do? They did not know anything about diets but they used herbs—they massaged the limbs with oils of juniper berries, fern extract, rosemary oil and linseed oil mixed in equal parts. They prepared the following herbs and boiled them in apple juice: willow bark, nettle, birch tree leaves, burdock root and primrose flowers. One cup three times daily.

They drank bitter water, which is lightly laxative in nature, and cleaned out their intestinal tract.

All of these above remedies have one goal. They take out waste material and/or stimulate the defense mechanism of your body so your metabolism jumps back to normal.

I want to share with you a recipe of Dr. Zabel, M.D., to determine when arthritis is true arthritis which means calcium deposits and an overacid condition; or when pains are due to something else like lack of calcium over alkalinity, metal or drug deposits or an overall toxic condition. Have your friend, wife, patient or child seated on a chair with their back to you. Over the bare skin run your two fingers lengthwise down the spine with a firm pressure three times. Then wait. If the red stripes are thin like pencil or the width of a finger and stay that way, pain is due to nerves. The redness will run broadly and sometimes like red hives when body tissue is toxic. It will take on an orange color when the pain is due to true arthritis—calcium deposits and an overacid condition.

Many medicines are extracted from herbs. Digitalis is a good example. The herbs are concentrated and the effective part is isolated and often combined with chemicals.

Whenever we use an herb without concentration or isolation, we employ a balancer and harmonizer. Herbs work on vibrations and bring harmony to disharmonic conditions by balancing out vibrations and re-establishing the delicate mineral households of the very cells.

Herbs furnish lots of trace minerals. For example, oatstraw is loaded with silicon, chamomile with calcium, sarsaparilla with hormones, etc.

The best way to take herbs is to take little sips frequently. Watermelon seed tea at the rate of one tablespoon per hour does more for the kidney than the drinking of six glasses a day would.

All herb leaves should be brewed and then allowed to steep for seven to ten minutes. All roots should be boiled. All seeds should be soaked in plenty of water and then heated. Just before the mixture boils, remove from heat and allow to cool.

Herbs never conflict with your physician's medicine. In fact, they help your medicine to be assimilated faster. Here are some time proven herbs you may want to hear about:

Flax seed tea is so soothing to an irritated digestive tract. It coats and heals and nourishes. Take two tablespoons of flax seed to one quart of water. Simmer for twenty minutes, strain and drink one cup of the warm mixture every two hours. For best results, alternate with carrot juice, one hour carrot juice, the next hour flax seed tea.

Peppermint is an alkalizer and a digestive aid.

Chamomile calms because of an extra amount of calcium which is in a form that the cells can readily make use of.

Fenugreek is grandma's mucous solvent. When mucous is accumulated in sinus, prostate, lungs, etc., this little seed surely goes to work.

Your liver may like the following herbal drink: One ounce **dandelion,** one ounce **horehound,** one-half ounce **sweet flag,** one ounce **flax seed** and one-half ounce **burdock.** Simmer in one quart water and take one ounce after meals.

Fresh **lemon** juice in a cup of hot water taken first thing in the morning will empty your gallbladder and start the day on a happy schedule.

Dr. Hohensee promoted the following formula for the eyes: Juices of one-half **potato,** one-half **onion** and one-quarter **green pepper.** Drink eight ounces of this one half hour before your supper and watch your eyes get clearer after thirty days.

Mistletoe softens muscles, bumps, fatty tumors, etc. and is a blessing for an overworked heart.

Blessed thistle tea is good for people who struggle with fever.

Break your smoking habits with **calamus, magnolia** and **myrtle** tea. Also chew **licorice.**

Sober up with **mullein leaf** tea.

Goldenseal is recommended for keeping young and it also takes away canker sores.

For sleeplessness try **hops, catnip, skullcap, black cohosh** and, if possible, **nerve root.** Taken in tea or capsules, it nourishes and balances the sleep center in your brain.

The **potassium herbs** are always very healing. They are chamomile, comfrey, fennel, mullein, nettle and walnut leaves.

Phosphorus herbs are good nerve coordinators and brain food. They include sunflower seeds, anise, fenugreek, watercress and chickweed.

Calcium herbs are chamomile, coltsfoot, horsetail, plantain, watercress and willow.

In an old herb book I found the following recipe for dandruff. Boil a handful of **willow leaves,** strain and wash your hair and scalp in it. Put a little concoction aside and dampen the scalp every day a little. I was amazed over the results.

A wonderful tonic for your liver is right in your back yard. Take a small handful of **dandelion leaves,** place in a blender with cranberry juice and, after liquefying, take six ounces two times daily.

To reduce the danger of forming gallstones, our forefathers took one tablespoon **ivy** tea after each meal.

Old-time recipe for bleeding gums and breaking capillaries: Wash and cut six **lemons** in little pieces. Cover with one and one-half quarts water and bring to boil. Turn off the heat and let sit for twenty-five minutes. Strain and set aside until cool. Take six ounces two times daily for ten days. In case of bleeding gums, hold juice in your mouth also.

Protruding veins on your hands do not look too pretty. In order to ease them and in many cases erase them, this is what the old folks did. Feel on the back of your head. Three fingers wide off the upper rim of your ears you will feel small indentations. Press on the left side of the head only. It will hurt. Hold it for one minute two times daily and the miracle will happen. The protruding veins on your hand will disappear.

In Mexico peasants place **mashed raw tomatoes** on swollen glands and a physician in Israel does the same for swelling of all kinds in the head. After reading his book and in my desperation to help my own child with some kind of brain tumor, I wrapped her head in a mass of mashed raw tomatoes and changed it every six hours. After the fourth application the smell was so bad that the whole room had an odor like rotten eggs. After three days her severe headaches left and after seven days her senses came back. However, I had to throw all her bedding away. The smell had penetrated everything.

Exercise for prolapsed colon: Clasp your hands together and press thumbs about the middle of solar plexus. Stand erect and pull in as hard as you can. When you rise up, you take a deep breath. When you go down, you exhale. This will throw the muscles into their proper position. Do this exercise twice daily (five breaths is sufficient), continue for four to six weeks and you will straighten the prolapsed transverse colon.

Swelling on knees: This appears to be a pretty frequent suffering but other joints may be afflicted too. There is water accumulations which make walking painful and distressing. Dr. Kunzle of Switzerland recommends the following application: Grate raw cabbage finely and wrap in a cheesecloth (one layer). Secure ends so cabbage cannot escape. Or make a sack out of the cheesecloth large enough to cover the afflicted area. Fill with grated cabbage and apply to knee. Cover with cellophane and wrap a large towel around it. Every night make a new compress. Nothing spectacular will happen until after the third day.

Here is one report: Mrs. Bunn of Cheyenne, Wyoming said, "I wrapped my swollen knee in a cabbage poultice. After the first two nights I felt great relief and eagerly made a compress every night. On the fourth morning I woke up at 5 a.m. from a terrible smell in the room. It was so putrid and foul smelling that I thought hell had broken loose. I turned on the light and found it came from the compress. I removed the dripping wet, evil smelling cabbage and oh wonder! The swelling from my knee was gone. The cabbage had pulled out all the liquid and that rotten stuff was about to penetrate my mattress. I applied the poultice three more nights and never had trouble since.

Burns: Place the burned hand or area in ice water or cold water until all pain is gone. If it is a second-or third-degree burn and no physician is available, mix in your blender the following formula:

one-half cup wheat germ oil
one-half cup honey
as many comfrey leaves as it will take to make a thick paste
a pinch of lobelia

Apply at once to the burned area.

This recipe was given to me by an herbalist. He adapted it from a writing in a monastery from the Middle Ages. You also can store this ointment and have it handy when needed. It takes the pain out at once and new skin will form after the third day. Comfrey is a cell grower and makes new, clean, good cells grow in a jiffy. Honey is a detoxifier. Vitamin E in wheat germ oil is a healer and heals without scars. Lobelia takes the pain away.

Pus diseases: These are diseases of decaying cells—ulceration, acne, boils, eczema and psoriasis.

two quarts apple cider
eight teaspoons garlic, freshly mashed
one teaspoon horseradish, grated

Put herbs in cider, let stand in warm place for twelve hours. Remove to a cold place and let stand twelve hours. Strain and use one tablespoon four times daily, also outwardly.

Heavy Metals: From the Aztecs comes this recipe to counteract the accumulation of heavy metals in the body:

sweet sumac
uva ursi
goldenseal root

101

Liver: Great celandine is an excellent detoxifier for the liver. This herb is particularly used when eyes are involved, vision blurred and liver stuffed.

Old German flu remedy:

one ounce peppermint
one ounce elder flowers

Brew these in one and one-half pints boiling water and drink six ounces every half hour.

High blood pressure:

three oranges
two lemons

Cut into pieces. Boil in one quart of water for fifteen minutes. Then add two tablespoons of honey. Boil another ten minutes. Strain and drink six ounces three times daily before meals. (NOT FOR DIABETICS)

A. Your Friends, the Friendly Bacteria

The human body is cut out to manufacture, to a great extent, its own B vitamins and certainly will do so when we give it the following chance.

The healthy intestine is loaded with friendly bacteria. Without the help of these workers, assimilation of food would not be possible. People would die of autointoxication. A friendly environment is necessary for these little helpers to multiply and work. Milk sugar acts as food for the friendly bacteria and helps to maintain a proper acid-alkaline balance.

After a lifesaving dose of penicillin, etc., the unfriendly bacteria are removed but the friendly bacteria also die. We can easily help this situation by eating lots of yogurt and using milk sugar on it. Or, a much simpler and faster solution is to drink several bottles of acidophilus milk. To sweeten your intestine and change it to a friendly environment, the following recipe is very good, cheap and wholesome:

> eight ounces powdered buttermilk
> eight ounces nonfat milk powder
> two ounces pure fruit pectin
> add one quart water and one quart fresh buttermilk
> sweeten each cup with one teaspoon of milk sugar

Take two tablespoons of acidophilus milk four times daily and drink two quarts or more of the above drink for several days.

Food with preservatives cannot fully be broken down to complete utilization. Lots of friendly bacteria die under the strain. More and more unfriendly bacteria take over and autointoxication begins. Only a healthy intestinal tract can manufacture B-complex vitamins.

We put out hate and expect love.

Our hearts are filled with envy but we expect happiness and peace.

We use force and want harmony.

We act cruel and expect sympathy.

We eat lifeless food and expect health.

Truly we are blind, or are we retarded?

References

The Bible
Contact Healing by Rev. Dr. F.M. Houston, D.C.
Neue Erkenntnisse in der Naturheilbehandlung by Dr. A. Rosendorff,
    M.D.
Gesundheit und Kraft durch Krautergold by M. Lassee
Moderne Ernahrungstherapie by Dr. Rudolf French, M.D.
Food, Facts and Fallacies by Dr. Carlton Fredericks, Ph.D.
Brotherhood of the White Temple founded by Dr. M. Doreal,
    Ms.D.
Let's Eat Right to Keep Fit by Adelle Davis
Feel Like a Million by Cathrine Elwood
Get Well Naturally by Linda Clark
Helping Your Health with Enzymes by Carlson Wade
Blut und Safte Reinigung by Erich Rauch, M.D.
Naturheilkunde by Professor Brauchle, M.D.
Sein by Rev. Max Zimmer, Ph.D.
A Bipolar Theory of Living Processes by George W. Crile
The Nature Doctor by Dr. A. Vogel, M.D.
Mental and Elemental Nutrients by Dr. Pfeiffer
Van Nostrand's Scientific Encyclopedia, 4th Ed., 1968
International Encyclopedia of Chemical Science, 1964, by D. Van
    Nostrand
Aynna Veda System by Charaka
Herbal Cures of Duodenal Ulcer and Gallstones by Frank Roberts
Silent Spring by Rachel Carson
Krautergold by Dr. Selig

Books by Hanna

Ageless Remedies from Mother's Kitchen
You will laugh and be amazed at all that you can do in your own pharmacy, the kitchen. These time tested treasures are in an easy to read, cross referenced guide. (92 pages)

Allergy Baking Recipes
Easy and tasty recipes for cookies, cakes, muffins, pancakes, breads and pie crusts. Includes wheat free recipes, egg and milk free recipes (and combinations thereof) and egg and milk substitutes. (34 pages)

Alzheimer's Science and God
This little booklet provides a closer look at this disease and presents Hanna's unique, religious perspectives on Alzheimer's disease. (15 pages)

Arteriosclerosis and Herbal Chelation
A booklet containing information on Arteriosclerosis causes, symptoms and herbal remedies. An introduction to the product *Circu Flow.* (17 pages)

Cancer: Traditional and New Concepts
A fascinating and extremely valuable collection of theories, tests, herbal formulas and special information pertaining to many facets of this dreaded disease. (65 pages)

Cookbook for Electro-Chemical Energies
The opening of this book describes basic principles of healthy eating along with some fascinating facts you may not have heard before. The rest of this book is loaded with delicious, healthy recipes. A great value. (106 pages)

God Helps Those That Help Themselves
This work is a beautifully comprehensive description of the seven basic physical causes of disease. It is wholistic information as we need it now. A truly valuable volume. (270 pages)

Good Health Through Special Diets
This book shows detailed outlines of different diets for different needs. Dr. Reidlin, M.D. said, "The road to health goes through the kitchen not through the drug store," and that's what this book is all about. (90 pages)

Hanna's Workshop
A workbook that brings together all of the tools for applying Hanna's testing methods. Designed with 60 templates that enable immediate results.

How to Counteract Environmental Poisons
A wonderful collection of notes and information gleaned from many years of Hanna's teachings. This concise and valuable book discusses many toxic materials in our environment and shows you how to protect yourself from them. It also presents Hanna's insights on how to protect yourself, your family and your community from spiritual dangers. (53 pages)

Instant Herbal Locator
This is the herbal book for the do-it-yourself person. This book is an easy cross referenced guide listing complaints and the herbs that do the job. Very helpful to have on hand. (109 pages)

Instant Vitamin-Mineral Locator
A handy, comprehensive guide to the nutritive values of vitamins and minerals. Used to determine bodily deficiencies of these essential elements and combinations thereof, and what to do about these deficiencies. According to your symptoms, locate your vitamin and mineral needs. A very helpful guide. (55 pages)

New Dimensions in Healing Yourself
The consummate collection of Hanna's teachings. An unequated volume that complements all of her other books as well as her years of teaching. (155 pages)

Old Time Remedies for Modern Ailments
A collection of natural remedies from Eastern and Western cultures. There are 20 fast cleansing methods and many ways to rebuild your health. A health classic. (115 pages)

Parasites: The Enemy Within
A compilation of years of Hanna's studies with parasites. A rare treasure and one of the efforts to expose the truths that face us every day. (62 pages)

The Pendulum, the Bible and Your Survival
A guide booklet for learning to use a pendulum. Explains various aspects of energies, vibrations and forces. (22 pages)

The Seven Spiritual Causes of Ill Health
This book beautifully reveals how our spiritual and emotional states have a profound effect on our physical well being. It addresses fascinating topics such as karma, gratitude, trauma, laughter as medicine . . . and so much more. A wonderful volume full of timeless treasures. (142 pages)

Spices to the Rescue
This is a great resource for how our culinary spices can enrich our health and offer first aid from our kitchen. Filled with insightful historical references. (64 pages)